Disputing Doctors

The socio-legal dynamics
of complaints about
medical care

Disputing Doctors

The socio-legal dynamics of complaints about medical care

Linda Mulcahy

Open University Press
Maidenhead · Philadelphia

Open University Press
McGraw-Hill Education
McGraw-Hill House
Shoppenhangers Road
Maidenhead
Berkshire
England
SL6 2QL

email: enquiries@openup.co.uk
world wide web: www.openup.co.uk

and

325 Chestnut Street
Philadelphia, PA 19106, USA

First published 2003

A catalogue record of this book is available from the British Library

ISBN 0 335 21244 1 (pb)   0 335 21245 X (hb)

The Library of Congress data for this book has been applied for from the Library of
Congress

Typeset by RefineCatch Limited, Bungay, Suffolk
Printed in Great Britain by Biddles Limited, *www.biddles.co.uk*

Contents

Acknowledgements

This book comes about as a result of my long-standing interest in the dynamics of disputes between doctors and patients. Much of the research which has led to this book was conducted in collaboration with others. Special thanks go to Judith Allsop who has collaborated with me on many of the projects discussed in this book and has acted as a sounding board, mentor and most importantly a friend. My work has been enriched by her scholarship and generosity. Thanks also go to Marie Selwood for assisting me in the research conducted and helping to get the manuscript into shape. Her calm and professionalism has been in stark contrast to my panic and disorganization. Finally my thanks go to my family and to Richard, Martha-Marie, Carl and Sally who have sustained me during a difficult year.

1 Introduction

This book examines the socio-legal dynamics of disputes between doctors and those who complain about them. More specifically it considers what is at stake when a patient or their champion questions the judgement of a hospital doctor. The making of a complaint about medical work provides an example of consumer activism which has received little attention from academics. Despite this, the issues raised in complaints have currency across a range of contemporary debates relating to the nature of professional power, the dynamics of the doctor-patient relationship, the value of notions of rights and trust as mechanisms to bind our society and the impact of law on everyday behaviour. The arguments I make are underpinned by empirical studies of how doctors react to being held accountable for clinical decisions by patients, their relatives and friends. Many of the studies referred to are ones in which I have been directly involved over the past 15 years. The writing of this book has given me the opportunity to reflect on the big messages which have emerged from the data which I have collected from complainants, doctors and National Health Service (NHS) managers over this period.

In one sense complaints are out of the ordinary events. One of the reasons that they are so fascinating is that they reverse the normal order of the doctor-patient exchange. When service users voice their grievances it is they who seek to diagnose the cause of a problem and prescribe a remedy to alleviate it. Research suggests that complaints are relatively rare when compared to the incidence of medical mishap or dissatisfaction among patients and their relatives. But when looked at alongside the incidence of legal claims or complaints about general practitioners (GPs) it is clear that complaints about hospital doctors are an accurate indicator of the tensions which arise in doctor-patient encounters. Moreover, these disputes highlight broader issues of interest to sociologists, lawyers and policy analysts. They mobilize social support systems, highlight social cleavages and are argued in terms of general morality. Analysing disputes offers the possibility of greater insights into social relations and conflict and this in turn allows us to use them to understand the wider social and cultural worlds in which complaints about doctors are embedded. It allows us not only to see social relations in action but also to understand the cultural systems in which they occur. The study of complaints leads straight to key issues for social scientists such as norms and ideology, power, rhetoric and oratory, personhood and agency, meaning and interpretation.

The issues raised in this book are highly relevant to academic and policy debates about the purpose and success of regulation in the public sector. Unlike many other forms of regulation which are proactive, the regulation of doctors through complaints occurs on an *ad hoc* basis. This form of calling to account is prompted by those using the service rather than salaried regulators. In this sense complaints about doctors are a form of reactive regulation which operate as a type of safety valve. They can be used to bring to light poor practices which have not been revealed or dealt with by more proactive regulatory systems such as clinical audit, risk management and the external reviews of the Commission for Health Audit and Inspection. But, in common with other regulatory models, the overseeing of complaint handling by the state has been hotly contested. The medical profession has resisted state interference and the shift towards handing jurisdiction over complaint handling to NHS managers. This book explores the ways in which such resistance to external regulation has manifested itself in national debate and service-level practice, and what this tells us about the ability of formal rules to govern everyday practice.

Complaints have come to the forefront of public debate in a number of other ways in recent years. A number of public inquiries have been launched which have considered whether instances of mismanaged medical care should have come to light much earlier than they did. These highlight the ways in which formal regulation has failed and the ways in which complaints can easily be marginalized as an indicator of quality. The Shipman Inquiry raised questions of whether quality initiatives in the NHS can ever be successful when so much work is carried out in the community, often by sole practitioners. The Kent and Canterbury cervical smear scandal has prompted concern over the failings of quality management in a large-scale hierarchy. The inquiry into the deaths of babies with serious heart conditions at Bristol Royal Infirmary initiated debates about the constraints on 'whistle blowing'. Most recently, three independent inquiries have been set up by the Secretary of State to look into the medical mishaps and poor performance of four doctors which went unchecked for two decades. In all of these cases, colleagues or patients of those to whom blame is being attributed had voiced their dissatisfaction with aspects of the care being provided. What was it about their criticisms which made such input from service users so unpalatable to professionals and managers? What caused their grievances to be so easily undermined and marginalized? The findings of those inquiries which have been published at the time of going to press suggest that complaints are deserving of more attention and that complainants have a right to have their concerns taken more seriously. But have the conditions in which such poor performance was allowed to continue and grievances allowed to fester changed sufficiently to ensure that lay accounts of experts' work can be given legitimacy? Credible systems for managing responses to claims about mismanaged cases cannot operate in a vacuum and will only be effective if the needs and fears of all those who participate in complaints systems are taken into account by the architects of grievance procedures. I argue in this book that before we can move forward we need to reflect on what we know and don't know about what motivates patients, doctors and managers to behave in the ways they do.

Mind the gap!

It is a basic tenet of this book that the effective formation of policy and law is facilitated by an understanding of how human beings react to policy, rules and regulation, and that issues of social control are central to issues of social policy. Set within this context, the book aims to contribute to the development of theories about the dynamics of disputes. In particular, it seeks to examine how the different participants in disputes between doctors and patients construct their accounts and the identity work they undertake in the process of constructing their narratives. A key theme to emerge is that there is a systemic distortion of meaning in interactions between doctors, patients and – to a lesser extent – managers. Conceptions of what constitutes appropriate care are formulated in significantly different ways by each of the parties to a complaint. Rather than representing a shared reality, accounts of illness, treatment and mistakes can represent an array of quite distinct forms of reasoning and ideology.

It is also argued that complaints are more than just a challenge to the individual complained about. They pose a broader threat to all doctors since they help to prompt debate about what is considered to be appropriate behaviour and the degree of accountability that doctors owe to patients. The development of complaints procedures provides one example of how the medical profession has dominated such debates. Throughout the course of such discussions doctors have maintained power over defining what is appropriate and debate also highlights the ways in which the elite of the profession have policed definitional boundaries in order to shield their members from external regulation. To date, much of this activity has only been visible to the laity at national level. Such an approach provides an important context for the present study, but in this book the emphasis is on how such resistance also manifests itself at service level. Focusing on complaints allows consideration to be given to the various ways in which the elite develop collective coping strategies, mobilize support networks and organize social interactions within the medical group on a day-to-day basis. In short, the book aims to cast a spotlight on what Kagan calls a 'handful of trees in the murky, ever-growing and incredibly diverse rainforest of regulatory programmes' (Kagan 1984: 1).

The book also aims to shed light on a form of administrative justice which has received scant attention from mainstream legal scholars. While complaints systems are pervasive they remain underinvestigated (Mulcahy et al. 1996b). Academics and practising lawyers have paid little serious attention to such systems of redress and even less attention to the issue of the place of complaints within the regulatory state. Complaints have been left alongside the study of other internal reviews in the public sector as something of a poor relation in mainstream administrative law (Davis 1969; Birkinshaw 1985a; McAuslan 1985; Mulcahy et al. 1996b). The characterization of complaint systems as 'low-level' methods of handling grievances has meant that administrative lawyers interested in studying them are seen as 'descending' for the purpose of their perusal (Harlow and Rawlings 1998). Administrative law textbooks tend not to include chapters on complaints and where notice has been taken of them there has been a tendency to view them in the context of their relationship to other things, most notably legal claims (see e.g. Carrier and Kendall 1990; Harpwood 1994). It follows that most parts of the administrative justice system have an extremely low profile in the minds and priorities of those who have in the past shaped policy relating to dispute resolution (Partington 1997).

As well as indicating the conservative nature of much public law scholarship, this attitude reflects the judiciary's tendency to construe narrowly the gateways to administrative and public law (Craig 1994).[1] Emphasis has instead been placed by legal academics on: the appellate courts, their models of reasoning and adjudication (Hawkins 1992); the structure of such rule-making bodies; the rules themselves, rather than on the people who interpret and implement these rules; and comparisons between courts and tribunals. This approach is often considered justified because of the so-called 'radiating' effects of court decisions (Galanter 1983: 119; Mulcahy 1999). According to this view, judicial pronouncements have a direct influence on the way that service users and administrators handle similar cases in the future. The courts are seen as having a declaratory role or as bestowing a regulatory endowment which casts a shadow over all disputes or acts as an incentive to debate (Fuller 1978; Mnookin and Kornhauser 1979; Galanter 1983; Fiss 1984).

However, there is also an argument that those cases which proceed to formal adjudication are unrepresentative of the range of disputes which arise in the citizen's interface with state authority (Ison 1997). According to this view, the way in which complaints systems operate constitutes an important aspect of how justice is achieved and how conflict is managed in contemporary society. Moreover, while judicial review and other public law remedies are important in constitutional terms they may be irrelevant to most citizens who want to challenge the decisions of public servants (Sainsbury 1994). Empirical studies of decision making have demonstrated that the majority of official decisions in the legal system of the modern state are not made by the judiciary but by front-line workers, like doctors and NHS managers, whose decisions are rarely visible.[2]

Where am I taking you?

Research into complaints raises a number of abstract and particular questions about the relationships between the state, the medical profession and patients. How have doctors come to dominate the management of clinical complaints? To what extent has the state shown an interest in challenging clinical autonomy and self-regulation? How have the tensions between the state, the medical profession and patients been handled at national level? What do complainants want to achieve when they voice their grievances? How do doctors at service level respond to complaints? How do they respond to the expectation that they tackle complaints in partnership with administrators and managers? This book aims to answer these questions. It has eight chapters. Following on from this introduction, Chapter 2 considers the wider political context in which complaints need to be understood. It focuses on the ways in which the relationship between the state, the medical profession and patients has come to be framed and the arguments which have supported the emergence of a self-regulatory professional model. It concludes with a review of contemporary challenges to this dominant model such as those posed by the consumer movement. Set against this backdrop, Chapter 3 charts the development of the hospital complaints procedure and the ways in which the elite of the medical profession have reacted to national policies on complaints. The analysis provides a case study of the ways in which professional groups strive to insulate themselves, maintain expert status and retain social power. Chapter 4 seeks to place the study of complaints in the context of other phenomena with which they have a connection. The purpose of this book is not to provide an in-depth analysis of medical negligence or the range of other processes through which complaints about doctors have been managed. Instead it looks at how medical mishap, dissatisfaction with health care, complaints and medical negligence have come to be defined and how the connections between them are best conceptualized. The link to previous chapters is that these terms are not value neutral. Rather they are the product of language which reflects power relations and dominant ways of thinking.

The second half of the book considers how the macro-level theories contained in the first half play themselves out on a day-to-day basis in NHS hospitals. Using a range of studies conducted across the social sciences, it considers how those involved in the making and handling of complaints respond to the challenges presented by public disagreements. It is argued that as well as representing a challenge to individual doctors, complaints can be seen as a symbolic challenge to the medical group. This is because the very act of making a complaint implies that the complainant has the competence and knowledge to challenge expert medical work. Moreover, the making of a complaint provides the trigger for managerial interferences in the doctor-patient relationship. An understanding of these broader threats to the profession goes some way to explaining why elite medical groups have sought to persuade policy makers against the setting up of formal regulatory frameworks for complaint handling. It also explains why doctors handling complaints at service level react so strongly to them and seek to circumvent and avoid formal regulations governing their responses.

In Chapter 5 discussion revolves around the construction of complaint narratives by patients and those who care for them. The emphasis here is on the ways in which complainants seek to explain the impact of medical intervention on their lives. Patients and their relatives often make complaints at a time when they are ill or suffering from the after-effects of treatment or bereavement. Their accounts strive to demonstrate the importance of their grievance within their own social networks and for the broader community. In the course of telling their stories of harm, hurt and indignity, complainants root their accounts in moral and caring identities which form part of the justification for making a complaint. Their claims to common-sense morality and competent lay medical work emphasize their own value systems and provide alternative frameworks to those of doctors within which the notion of competence can be judged. By way of contrast, Chapter 6 focuses attention on the ways in which doctors respond to criticisms of their work. An appreciation of such responses to complaints allows us to understand why complaints procedures do not operate in the ways anticipated by bureaucrats and policy makers, and to explore whether the formal goals of constructive and conciliatory approaches to complaints are realistic or achievable. Doctors feel threatened by complaints and they are likely to have a severe emotional impact on those who receive them. The data discussed demonstrate that doctors tend to provide bio-medical explanations of the causes of complaints in which the language of consumerism and rights is noticeably missing. They also rely strongly on notions of collective medical identity in these accounts and achieve a reconstruction of their damaged sense of worth by deconstructing and undermining complainants' accounts. The final substantive chapter considers the role of managers in the handling of complaints. It looks at the extent to which they perceive their role to be to protect the interests of the patient population, their employees or the resources of the organization for which they work. Data are presented which suggest that managers are more likely than not to adopt a conciliatory approach towards doctors in the course of handling complaints but that, despite this, doctors continue to resist their intervention in the handling of complaints.

The book concludes with a final chapter which reflects on the data and discussion presented in earlier chapters. It is argued that the topic of complaints provides an insightful case study into the interface of law and medicine, science and art, and expert and lay narratives. More specifically it considers the ways in which the professional project of doctors is achieved on a day-to-day basis. Despite the attraction of rights discourse to consumer groups it is concluded that, for doctors, legal regulation and being held to account is seen as an oppressive force in the doctor-patient relationship. Like the stories of illness and treatment provided by complainants, the rights discourse which is increasingly encouraged by policy makers presents a radically different picture of entitlement and obligation from that employed within medicine. All of these different discourses make claims to morality and use of the rhetoric of communitarianism. But what is most obvious are the limitations of law and the rhetoric of rights when placed within an alien culture.

All change?

During the course of this book being written the government has expressed a strong commitment to reforming both the clinical negligence and complaints systems. It seems likely that renewed thought will be given to the advantages of a no-fault compensation scheme for clinical negligence claims and that an extra degree of independence will be introduced in the handling of appeals against the initial reaction to complaints at service level. These initiatives are undoubtedly important and will provide a slightly different context for future work, but as my work has progressed and come to fruition I have come to realize that the relevance of the empirical studies reported here is not that they relate specifically to a particular system but rather that large themes emerge from across systems. Much of the second half of the book concentrates on a micro-level analysis of particular complaints, allegations and stories. The signals which these analyses send are that the tensions inherent in the handling of individual complaints reflect the political debate which occurs between politicians, bureaucrats and the elite of the profession at national level about the appropriate role of doctors in our society. The stories told by complainants, doctors and managers are tales of boundaries and expectations. These dynamics do not change with new procedures, they just operate in a slightly different context. The narratives I unravel in this book take place within a context of normative frameworks and cultural assumptions which change much more slowly. While processes for the resolution of disputes can change rapidly, the dynamics of the doctor-patient relationship are much slower to respond.

Notes

1   It may also be explained by the fact that many studies of complaints procedures have been empirical and that some public lawyers have afforded such studies lower academic status. McAuslan (1985), for instance, refers to the distinction between high and low constitutional theory, placing empiricists in the latter category.

2   The emphasis placed on more formal attempts at grievance resolution at the top of the civil justice hierarchy has not gone unnoticed. A handful of writers have made attempts to put complaints on the research agenda and the work of the 'Sheffield School' is particularly worthy of note (Birkinshaw 1985a, 1985b; Lewis et al. 1987; Seneviratne and Cracknell 1988; Lewis and Birkinshaw 1993; Seneviratne 1994). This book represents a modest attempt to redress this imbalance.

2   All the president's men

The relationships between the state, the medical profession and doctor-patient disputes

Introduction

The challenge to doctors posed by complaints cannot be fully understood without reference to the role played by medical professionals in wider society. Doctors wield considerable power based on their social status, economic wealth and unique access to, and control of, a body of knowledge which is highly valued by society and the state. Their claim to power is based on the notion that medics possess a rarefied knowledge which can be used for the good of society. Their contention that their knowledge is scientific and rational endows their accounts of events with a generalizability and rationality which compares with the less cherished subjective and anecdotal accounts of patients. Access to a discourse of science has brought considerable political strength to the profession and has allowed doctors to claim considerable professional autonomy. This chapter considers the role that the state has played in promoting the legitimacy of these claims and the profession's largely unfettered jurisdiction over complaint handling which has come about as a result. It explores how the boundaries of what can be challenged through complaints have been drawn by the state, interest groups and the profession. It looks at how expectations of accountability held by the profession have emerged and become reinforced by the state. Significantly, the relatively recent emergence of formal complaint procedures reflects a diminution of professional autonomy which has been made possible since the emergence of the NHS, and more recently by the rise of managerial authority within it. Subsequent chapters explore how particular complaint systems have come into being. This chapter allows such developments to be contextualized by exploring the broader political climate in which this was made possible.

Doctors' authority in society and within the medical consultation depends on an acceptance of their power and the legitimacy of medical discourse. When patients call doctors to account by questioning their judgement they lay claim to an alternative interpretation of circumstances, they step out of 'the sick role' anticipated of them. In many accounts, claim is made to an expertise which contrasts with, and threatens, the scientific basis of knowledge claimed by the doctor. At one level, a discrete complaint can be seen as a mere request for information or a fuller explanation. Cumulatively, complaints, and the rapid rise in their incidence, can be seen as a fundamental challenge to claims of knowledge.

But despite the fact that external regulation of medical work appears to have increased significantly during the last century, the medical profession has continued to be extremely successful in claiming jurisdiction over its work and, more specifically, over the handling of complaints. The principle of self-regulation has proven to be a convenient one for both state and profession. Viewed from the perspective of the profession, it has allowed it to attain considerable social closure by leaving it the freedom, at both a collective and individual level, to determine what constitutes appropriate treatment and behaviour. This high level of autonomy has been justified on a number of grounds. The profession has argued that doctors should be judged by other doctors in a system of self-regulation with maximum clinical autonomy, and this view remains influential. In such self-regulatory models, expert workers control the delivery of a service *and* complaint handling. Self-regulation is seen as the only appropriate form of control when criticisms are lodged because only the experts themselves have the ability and information to judge the competence of a colleague. It is no coincidence then that certain professional groups, most notably medicine and law, have been able to self-regulate in areas of work where extensive training is necessary to acquire a high degree of specialist knowledge and expertise. Typically, the application of this knowledge requires not only technical skill, but also the exercise of expert judgement within a personal service. The professions also argue that the public is best served by groups which are independent of state control. It is claimed that outside interference in this process would undermine a profession's public orientation and subject it to external regulation that would be harmful to both the profession and the public interest.

It is not just in the UK that such arguments prevail. All economically advanced societies have special forms of regulation for professional groups. The claims made by medics have been attractive to successive governments because they allow for the devolution of responsibility for, and the costs of, regulation to the medical profession, while providing a persuasive rationale for doing so (Stacey 1992). Harrison et al. (1990) have viewed the arrangement as an example of liberal corporatism, a process through which the state eases its own problems in managing society by offering favours and status to a few selected interest groups in return for their agreement to behave in 'moderate' ways. They have argued that 'The big deals [are] worked out between the state and "the peak associations" (the favoured, elite, organized groups) and then "sold" to the rank and file and general public' (1990: 23).

Viewed in this way it can be seen that the needs of state and profession are symbiotic. Barbara Castle and Richard Crossman's diaries testify to the fact that in the British tradition of government medical elites continue to be in close and constant contact with ministers and government officials (Crossman 1977; Castle 1980). In this way, politicians have sought to resolve disagreement by the incorporation of interest groups in the process of decision making prior to the announcement of policy goals (Klein 1989).[1]

But it is important to note that the granting of such powers to the profession has been far from unpopular. Kelleher et al. (1994) argue that the appeal of a strong medical profession has been fuelled by rising concern about public health, the decline of organized religion, the development of pharmacological products, the growth of research laboratories and the increasing confidence in science. Medical work has been particularly highly valued in times of war and epidemics, and even in peaceful and healthy conditions the public has been keen to be protected from 'quacks'. It has also been argued that the development of professional power based on skill was an attractive alternative to a society in which the attainment of economic and social standing was largely dependent on class during the nineteenth century. In his impressive treatise on the rise of professional society, Perkin (1996: 9) argues that the ideal of a society in which hierarchy was determined by expertise was seductive because it suggested their power was attainable by the disadvantaged: 'The ideal . . . implied a principle of social justice which extended to the whole population the right to security of income, educational opportunity, decent housing in a clean environment and, some professionals would say, the right and obligation to work'.

Significantly, the political position enjoyed by patient groups is not the same as that enjoyed by the medical profession, a factor which has lead Klein (1989) to label patients as the 'ghosts' of the NHS. The relative absence of patient voices has meant that the NHS has been allowed to develop in a particular way without reference to the authentic views and critiques of those receiving its services. The emphasis in political debate about health services has, until relatively recently, been on public accountability through political process rather than public participation. When these processes failed to check spreading professional power it was hoped that managers would be able to mediate the tensions between lay and professional groups which might emerge. But inquiries such as those at Ely Hospital in Cardiff and more recently the Bristol Royal Infirmary (Bristol Inquiry 2001) have provided a salutary reminder that the interests of patients are not always protected by managers who may be more concerned about their relationships with staff. In his discussion of negotiations about the setting up of the NHS, Willcocks (1967) suggested that from its early years onwards politicians and professionals laid claim to the ability to determine what was in the public interest although what resulted could often be seen as cover or justification for the promotion of their own self-interests. The absence of authentic consumer views in the journals, articles and official reports which chart the history of the NHS can also be explained by the lack of consumer organizations to put their views forward. Even where groups have formed, patient organizations face the problem that their presence is bound to be less rooted in the political consciousness than established professional bodies. To be a doctor and represent medical views is to represent a continuing group, but to be fit and represent the transient population of patients is much more difficult.

Recent commentators have reminded us that in a liberal democracy the expectation is that the medical profession's compact with the state brings with it an obligation not to abuse this asymmetry of expertise. In other words, self-regulation only works while the profession is trusted. In the words of the *Report of the Public Inquiry into Children's Heart Surgery at Bristol Royal Infirmary 1984–95*:

> The purpose of the system of regulation must be to assure the public of the competence of healthcare professionals and, when necessary, to protect them. As such it needs the widest involvement of professionals, of the principal employer and of the public. It cannot achieve its purpose if it is a system which is designed and operated solely by particular professionals for their professional peers. Nor can it achieve its purpose if it is solely a matter for employers within the NHS. An effective system of professional regulation must be owned collectively. Further, it needs an independence from the professions and from government which allows it to act in the public interest.
>
> (Bristol Inquiry 2001, para 201)

When the power wielded by a group becomes visible it is increasingly common for there to be calls to regulate it in some way in order to render the group more accountable to wider society. What constitutes a satisfactory regulation policy is culturally specific, shifts over time and varies according to the perspective of the stakeholders involved. It is influenced by such abstract ideas as efficacy, value, cost and social justice. I suggest that recent claims by patient groups that clinical complaint handling should be more intensively regulated reflects a crisis of confidence among consumers which has caused the elite of the profession to mobilize resistance to the call for greater accountability. For some this mirrors wider changes in society. Discussing trust in the context of the Shipman Inquiry, O'Neill (2002) suggested in her Reith lectures that 'loss of trust' has indeed become a cliché of our times. The study of complaints has much to contribute to our understanding of this statement within an NHS context. The tensions reflected in and created by complaints do much to reveal how experts and the laity conceptualize the doctor-patient relationship and the limits of trust. Calls for increases in consumer participation in complaint systems can be seen as threatening the delicate balance between state regulation and self-regulation, and between clinical autonomy and managerial or consumer interference in medical work.

How has self-regulation been achieved?

Throughout the course of the history of the medical profession it has been important for medical groups to have their identity and work recognized and licensed; first by the established Church and more recently by the state. The most important aspect of such recognition is not merely that it gave the right to practise to those within a recognized group but that it prohibited those outside the group from practising. This has been achieved most easily by focusing on education and class. The majority of legislative activity has emphasized the need to ensure that doctors are adequately educated and for much of the history of the profession this has meant that they must also have a substantial income.[2] Such statutes were passed after long campaigns fought by practitioners keen to achieve social closure. One of the most important recognition exercises took place in the mid-nineteenth century with the formal recognition of the General Medical Council (GMC).[3]

Stacey (1992) has argued that the establishment of the GMC was a crucial part of the profession's collective upward mobility but, significantly, this was achieved at the expense of other organizations. At the end of the nineteenth century, 22 licensing bodies accredited doctors and it was not until the Medical Registration Act of 1858 led to the establishment of the GMC that licensing was undertaken by one centralized body.[4] The make-up of the new GMC, drawn from corporations of physicians, surgeons and apothecaries, reflected a far from united group of practitioners, and intra-professional rivalry between the different specialists was rife. But collectively they gained a considerable amount by protecting their professional autonomy and in exercising their powers were subject only to review by the Privy Council, which could reverse their decisions.

The Act of 1858 granted powers to restrict entry to the profession but also imposed obligations on the GMC. It charged it with the responsibility to compile a single register of medical practitioners qualified to a level recognized by them.[5] In addition, they were required to discipline recalcitrant members whose standard of practice was poor, and had the power to take away the licences of such practitioners. Parry and Parry (1976) have suggested that the ability of powerful groups within the profession to negotiate this power was largely due to the fact that medics had become an organized pressure group prior to the entry of the state into the formerly private field of health care.

While the state was progressively becoming more centrally involved in the practice of medicine, through its operation of policies relating to the Poor Law and public health, there was until 1919 no central state agency dealing with complaints and poor performance other than the GMC.[6]

It followed that, by the time discussions about the setting up of the NHS began, the medical profession had an established and authoritative political voice in negotiations between the profession and the state. For many historians, the NHS Act of 1946 owed much more to the long discussions between the profession and the Minister of Health about channels of command and the degree of regulation than it did to any doctrinaire ideals of the governing Labour Party (Willcocks 1967; Cartwright 1977; Klein 1989). The reliance the state placed on the support of the profession is aptly reflected in the Chancellor of the Exchequer's plea in the House of Commons that lengthy debate was essential when dealing with a great and honourable profession. The general consensus from government was that policy should be settled by negotiation and achieved with the utmost goodwill (Cartwright 1977). As Harrison et al. have argued: 'The NHS was founded on a complicated bargain between several parties most notably the government, which brought to bear both money and powers of legislation, and doctors, with resources of monopoly, expertise and popular esteem' (1990: 1).[7]

Even the emergence of a welfarist approach to the provision of health care posed threats and presented opportunities for doctors. On the one hand, doctors were offered secure and regular payment and use of state-funded facilities. Politicians also promised a more rational and better-funded approach to health care than had been the case in the past.[8] On the other, there was the potential for them to be subjected to closer scrutiny and the British Medical Association (BMA) expressed strong concerns that professional freedom was at risk.[9] The profession was particularly fearful of a suggestion that the new health service should come under the control of local authorities in order to build on their experience of managing the existing municipal hospitals.[10] Rather than submit to such a 'bureaucratic' model based on accountability to elected politicians, the BMA favoured a model where policy and central organization would be undertaken by a body divorced from day-to-day political control and largely under the control of fellow medics. Their aim was to achieve as great a measure of executive decentralization as possible.

In the eventual deal negotiated by the profession and policy makers, there were concessions on both sides but the medical profession fared particularly well. This conclusion has led Cartwright (1977) to surmise that Bevan was not the great architect of the NHS of the popular imagination but much more akin to a jobbing builder who happened to get some of his tender accepted. The original unified and centralized administrative model envisaged by politicians floundered because of medical opposition and gave way instead to separate specialist administrations.[11] The NHS remained in reality three separate organizations which dealt with secondary care, primary care and community services, with separate administrative and complaints structures to deal with each.[12] In the words of Willcocks, it was 'Split rather than unified, free but with private practice and including both elective and appointed systems: all in all an odd administrative structure, especially when viewed against early attempts at a simplified but comprehensive administration' (1967: 19–20).

The profession also negotiated the addition of clinical authority to the principles of comprehensiveness, universality and collectivism favoured by the Labour government of the time as the appropriate foundations for a national health service. Teaching hospitals, which were generally managed by the elite of the profession, were accorded a special status and independence not accorded to other hospitals. Perhaps most significantly, medics secured representation on governing bodies at regional and local level and remained almost completely in control of decisions as to what care should be offered to patients.[13] Such influence was not offered to other NHS health professionals such as nurses or, indeed, to other professionals such as teachers who were also involved in discussions about a radically reformed public education service. Bevan later famously described how, in his dealings with the medical profession, he had 'stuffed their mouths with gold' (Stacey 1988: 45).[14]

Consensus was not without its cost within the profession which remained divided on a number of issues. The BMA's own first plan of the shape of a national health service launched in 1942 was followed by alternative plans drawn up by medical groups such as that produced by the Socialist Medical Association. Moreover, the joint representative committee of the profession appointed to negotiate NHS policy with the government undoubtedly had what the BMA considered to be a troublesome fringe (Willcocks 1967) and the Royal Colleges, Society of Medical Officers, Medical Practitioners Union and Socialist Medical Association often put forward different viewpoints. These rifts forced the BMA to conduct a referendum of members' views on the idea of an NHS and drove a particularly noticeable wedge between hospital consultants and GPs. Seeing that he could not satisfy all constituents, Bevan deliberately encouraged such rifts and sought to gain the support of the most influential parts of the profession.[15] The result was that a negotiated settlement was achieved but the damage done to intra-professional politics was considerable and apparent for many decades to come. GPs lost the right to sell the goodwill of their practice and to work whenever it suited them. Their work also came under the administrative control of new executive councils, which operated as their paymasters and were made up of equal numbers of the profession and laity.[16] Moreover, these councils were given the power to establish special committees to hear complaints about doctors who failed to fulfil certain terms of their contract. As the GMC had established disciplinary powers over all doctors since 1858, this particular measure set in place an alternative system of grievance procedures for some patients, a model which in time was to pro-liferate across sectors. This resulted in a confusing web of complaints and disciplinary systems which served and continues to serve to confuse patients wanting to voice a formal grievance.

The bargain struck by the government of the day and the medical profes-sion has remained resilient and resulted in the medical profession being closely involved and consulted about the management of the NHS over sub-sequent decades. In the words of one commentator: 'Above all, the medical profession has made sure that governments, whatever their ideology or ambi-tions, would think long and hard before seeking to change the structure of the NHS in any way which would bring the underlying concordat with the medical profession into question' (Klein 1989: 57). Rather than undermining professional influence, commentators such as Klein (1989) have argued that subsequent reforms served to expand further the representation of doctors throughout the NHS. In his view, the NHS became festooned with professional advisory committees and the voice of the expert became set in concrete in the institutional structure much more firmly than in 1946. For him the real polit-ical battle in the health care arena has been a definitional one of whether or not specific problems or issues are labelled 'medical'. According to his thesis, the institutionalization of a medical voice at all levels of the NHS has allowed doctors to medicalize management. The elite of the profession continues to make a contribution to policy making within the NHS Executive and Depart-ment of Health (DoH) and through their consultative machinery. Their views are also heard through membership of regional offices of the NHS Executive and health authorities have access to medical advice from doctors working in hospitals and on medical advisory and local medical committees. Finally, NHS Trusts include a medical director on their board and rely extensively on advice from their medical staff (Ham 1992).

The acceptance of the principle of widespread medical autonomy carried the 'seeds of future problems' for those concerned about holding doctors to account (Allsop 1995: 33). As the NHS developed, the profession continued to protect the privileges it had negotiated for its members and resisted continued attempts to rein in its power (Perkin 1996). Numerous examples of this ten-dency exist which serve to reflect the extent of the profession's continued influence. Subsequent attempts to transfer responsibility for health policy to local government in the 1970s, for instance, were debated by both the Labour and Conservative Parties but were eventually considered unfeasible because the medical profession expressed such strong opposition. The government was compelled to be satisfied with a realigning of some health authority boundar-ies with those of local authorities instead. Professional groups within the NHS have also generally fared better than others in terms of pay increases although they set the precedent of striking in order to achieve this in the 1970s (Harrison et al. 1990).

Managerial interference with medical work was also long resisted. The Cogwheel working party (Ministry of Health 1967) attempted to promote a managerial consciousness in the medical profession, but marginal success was eventually achieved only through a revised strategy of persuasion rather than imposition. More recently, attempts to encourage doctors into management have proved unsuccessful and suggest that a tribal culture still exists, despite widespread support for cooperation between managers in the influential Griffiths Report (DHSS 1983b).

The cooperation of the profession in launching new initiatives has also been crucial to policy developments. Allsop (1995) has charted how the medical profession's resistance to change resulted in negotiations relating to the 1974 reorganization of the service taking ten years to complete and an eventual compromise of interests in favour of the profession. Moreover, Stacey (1992) draws attention to how the Merrison Committee, set up to inquire into the operation of the GMC in 1975, was specifically instructed by the government, under pressure from elite members of the medical profession, not to examine whether professional regulation worked. Stacey argues that, as a consequence, nothing in the resulting report provides a check on the GMC's tendency to pay more attention to the interests of the profession than to the needs of complainants.

Challenges to the profession

The growth of political, social, cultural and economic power in the medical profession has not gone unchecked. As well as enjoying its achievements, the profession has also suffered certain crises of credibility which have affected its ability to argue for the legitimacy of clinical autonomy and self-regulation (Kelleher et al. 1994). Commentators have charted a number of ways in which confidence in the willingness of the profession to moderate the behaviour of poorly performing doctors can be measured. Among these are the occasional crises and scandals about mismanaged care and inadequate monitoring of work which the current president of the GMC has described as having sapped the self-confidence of the profession (Catto 2002: 4). Perkin (1996) cites, for example, a spate of 'scandals' in which doctors would not give evidence against medical colleagues in malpractice suits, a number of widely publicized drug abuse cases involving GPs and at least one notorious case of a forensic pathologist convicted of rigging legal evidence. More recent examples of such scandals include investigations into the activities of Dr Peter Elwood undertaken by the CHI, the investigation of allegations of indecent assault made against Dr Peter Green, the inquiry into the practices of Dr Harold Shipman, and, of course, the inquiry into heart surgery at Bristol Royal Infirmary. It is significant that many of these investigations have detected the presence of an NHS culture in which complaints were not listened to or analysed.[17] These inquiries have attracted media coverage, pressure group activity and political concern and, in some cases, have created a significant impetus for change (Ham 1992). Inquiries and investigations into systemic mismanagement of risk and poor practice continue to provide windows of opportunity in which the government can press for more radical mechanisms for accountability than might normally be possible in their negotiations with the profession (Rosenthal et al. 1999). It is clear that public outrage remains an important bargaining tool in the ongoing negotiations between state and profession.

Recent years have also witnessed an increasing emphasis on managerial control of medical work and the political will to steer the NHS in the direction of bureaucratic or legal models of regulation has been much more apparent than in the early years of the NHS. The role of all professional groups has shifted with industrial maturity, and changes to their work pattern and identity have been particularly evident in the post-Fordist era. Writing in the context of health, Harrison et al. (1990) have argued that there has been a very distinct movement from a scenario of medical 'professional monopolists' to one where a strong challenge is being mounted from managerial corporate rationalizers. Recent reforms have heralded a new wave of managerialism which could be viewed as another instance of antagonistic threats to the collective integrity of the profession. For some commentators the less deferential approach to all professions witnessed in recent decades marks the return of ideology into the policy framework.[18] Perkin (1996) argues that this new approach to professionals was particularly obvious during the 'spontaneous attacks' which Margaret Thatcher and her political colleagues made on the three ancient professions of law, medicine and the clergy, fuelled by their belief that the extensive power wielded by these groups encouraged inertia in the provision of services. Her vision was of public services with a strong centre and strong leadership at service level, with the role of intermediaries in the middle, such as the medical profession, reduced. Harrison and Pollitt (1994) have also noted that in their drive for a return to market principles and increased efficiency, Conservative governments in the 1980s and 1990s tended to perceive professionals in the NHS as obstacles rather than allies. The era was one in which doctors were forced to defend their claims to restrictive practices in the name of clinical autonomy. Managerial influence was enhanced at the direct expense of the profession (Klein 1989). Historically, such regulation has been most notable in initiatives involving the management of budgets.[19] More recently, managers have gradually been able to exert more control over the activities of doctors by means of such mechanisms as improved information systems and clinical budgeting.

One of the most far-reaching changes to systems of accountability in the NHS came in the form of the introduction of the NHS and Community Care

Act in 1990. This legislation allowed the Thatcher government to challenge the power of medical professionals by strengthening the NHS management structure (Allsop and Mulcahy 1996). It gave managers unprecedented powers to take part in the appointment of hospital consultants, negotiate their job plans and participate in decisions about which doctors should receive distinction awards. A past president of the Royal College of Physicians has suggested that this is particularly relevant when looked at in the context of poor performance. He has argued that:

> the competitive marketing philosophy of the 'new' NHS has introduced the need to improve outcome figures for medical intervention and, hence, to eliminate incompetence and inefficiency; the strengthening of managerial systems has given administrators the teeth to take action against a doctor whose performance appears not to match that of his colleagues.
>
> (Hoffenberg 1995: xi)

Two important new forms of management developed as a result of these reforms. On the one hand, a number of organization-wide systems (such as quality, risk, performance, bed management, tighter controls over hospital consultants' contracts),[20] were introduced and merit awards reformed, so that rewards and credit were based on clinical skills and commitment to management.[21] At the same time, complaints procedures were renewed more frequently during this period than at any other time in the history of the NHS. New structures were also introduced within medicine to manage areas of clinical activity, such as management through clinical directorates and clinical protocols (Berwick et al. 1992a, 1992b). Such developments have led to claims that medicine is being de-professionalized as part of a more general trend of rationalization and the codification of expert knowledge (Haug 1973, 1988; Haug and Lavin 1983) or even proletarianized in line with the requirements of advanced capitalism (McKinlay and Stoekl 1988). New supra-regulatory frameworks have also emerged in recent years to challenge self-regulatory structures. The National Clinical Assessment Authority (NCAA),[22] National Institute for Clinical Excellence (NICE), Commission for Health Audit and Inspection (CHAI) and National Patient Safety Agency have taken on responsibility for assuring the quality and safety of patient care. Changes of this kind have become so common that Klein was moved to remark as far back as 1989 that 'The secret garden of professional autonomy seemed to be shrinking to the size of a window box' (1989: 102).

Inter-professional rivalries have also played their part in undermining the power of the medical profession. Kelleher et al. (1994) argue, for instance, that the nursing elite have been embarking on a process of occupational development which has forced a redefinition of the relationship between medicine and nursing (see also Dingwall et al. 1988). It is certainly true that nurses have been more prepared to take on managerial roles than doctors and many have veered towards quality management roles. But the advent of nurse consultants and nurse practitioners has made it clear that, in addition, nurses are prepared to challenge the traditional clinical territory of doctors. Those professionals who work alongside doctors have been strategically placed to observe the skills of doctors and determine the extent to which their knowledge base is esoteric and rarefied – as has been claimed. Lupton (1997) has also drawn attention to the challenge posed by the number of patients turning to complementary or alternative medicine, and Saks (1994) has charted the growth of complementary medicine as a direct attack on the bio-medical model of care. Interest in alternatives may be explained in a number of ways: as part of the disillusionment many people feel with the dehumanizing effects of 'scientific' medicine; the manifest lack of interest that doctors display in treating them as people; or the failure of modern medicine to match up to expectations. Klein comments that even by the 1970s 'A stage where once the leaders of the medical profession had been able to soliloquize with little interruption had now become crowded with actors all clamouring to be heard' (1989: 82).

Intra-professional rivalries within the medical profession have also had a part to play in the diminution of respect for medics. Disputes between different professional groups are nothing new, indeed they are a key feature of historians' accounts of the growth of medical power (see, e.g. Willcocks 1967; Cartwright 1977). The structural divisions between primary, secondary and public health are particularly significant since each group enjoys a different relationship with the state and their interests are often far from synonymous. But recent decades have seen more organized resistance to the elite of the profession. The 1970s was a particularly interesting period in this regard. An increased militancy among NHS staff about their terms and conditions of employment led to something of a convergence between the tactics of trade unions and professional medical organizations. Not only did doctors take industrial action for the first time, but the BMA (which had been granted sole negotiating rights on pay and conditions) was directly challenged by the Medical Practitioners Union and the Hospital Consultants and Specialists Association (HCSA) regarding its claim to speak for the whole of the profession. More recently, the same claim has been made by the Hospital Consultants and Specialists Association in relation to negotiations over pay and contracts (HCSA 2002). Political ideology has also had a part to play in these rifts. The Socialist Doctors Association has often been in opposition to the BMA and unions representing NHS staff have regularly questioned the efficacy of consultants seeing some patients in private beds in NHS hospitals. Conflicts of interest based on seniority and gender have also become apparent. The Junior Hospital Doctors' Association, formed in 1966, has worked to end the large differential in pay between junior doctors and hospital consultants, and the Medical Women's Federation seeks to support women doctors and undermine sexism within the profession. These divisions suggest that there are considerable weaknesses in professional corporatism, leading some observers to remark that the reality is more akin to anarchic syndicalism (Klein 1989).

Challenges to medical power from the laity have also had some impact on their political power. Until recent times, there was relatively little opposition to the traditional medical view of patients as the passive recipients of medical care. It was widely accepted that doctors should decide what treatment was necessary and determine how much a patient needed to know about their condition. Such paternalistic attitudes were justified in the interests of patient welfare and by reference to the Hippocratic oath (Teff 1994). In recent decades patients have begun to assert that they have the right to be more involved in their treatment, and to be better informed.[23] The development of a consumer movement has also been symbiotic with the growth in media coverage of doctors and a tendency for the media to be more critical of them (Kelleher et al. 1994). In particular the media have given more extensive coverage to the failings of medicine and the mistakes made by doctors. In the words of Lupton, 'As in the United States and Britain, media representations of the medical profession in Australia have veered from portraying doctors as the saint-like saviour of lives or restorer of good health (particularly if they are surgeons), to criticizing doctors for medical negligence, avarice and sexual harassment' (1997: 483).

Some have argued that the media's role in the transformation of views about the medical profession rarely gets the attention or credit it deserves (Strong 1983). Not only has press coverage of health matters increased but so too have the use of lay, as opposed to medical, perspectives (Kelleher et al. 1994). Ham (1992) cites the example of television coverage of 'Cinderella' services – such as the reporting of the abuses at Rampton Special Hospital in the 1970s – as an example of this. He argues that, at times, journalists and television producers have taken on the mantle of pressure groups for underprivileged sections of the community. All these factors are seen to contribute to an erosion of the traditional power of doctors, an increase in their economic vulnerability and alienation in the medical workforce (Lupton 1997). This development has in turn empowered readers, listeners and viewers to think about how medical decision making might be challenged.

The medical profession has not remained immune from these pressures. The publication of the DoH's consultation paper on the reform of the GMC in May 2002 heralded the introduction of radical changes to make the GMC more accountable and better able 'to meet the requirements society places on regulatory bodies' (GMC 2002: 1). Changes in the revalidation of doctors, a simplification and review of the fitness to practise framework and a reform of the structure, constitution and governance of the GMC to allow for more involvement of lay members have followed. In recent years, the GMC has also expanded the range of its activities in relation to both promoting good practice and identifying poor practice. In the case of the former, what the competent doctor should do has been spelt out in increasing detail. In the case of the latter, the health procedures introduced by the GMC put in place a mechanism for dealing with doctors who are identified as 'at risk' of causing medical mishaps. Once identified, they can be offered treatment and support. A new appraisal scheme introduced in April 2001 to give doctors regular feedback on their performance is also being implemented. Finally, new revalidation schemes requiring doctors to demonstrate on a five-yearly cycle that they remain up to date and fit to practise were steered through Parliament in 2002.

Conclusion

This chapter has attempted to place the challenge of complaints within a political and social context. It has explored the connections between the state, the medical profession and patients and suggested that expectations about their relationships are in a constant state of flux and negotiation. The expectations of all these stakeholders have changed considerably over time, and changes in the balance of power and responsibility have been particularly noticeable since the inception of the welfare state. The hiving off of responsibility for regulating medical work has been an attractive option for politicians. But the compact between state and profession which was agreed has resulted in a mixed regulatory model in which the state provides a framework of accountability but relinquishes control over the details to the medical profession.[24] However, an acceptance of welfarism and more interventionist policies as the more appropriate form of governance in the latter half of the twentieth century served to challenge the validity of the compact between state and profession. Medical power and medical discourses have also been challenged by the growth of consumerism, of which complaining is one aspect. Consumerism has manifested itself in many other ways in the media, in political campaigning and in the increased use of the courts, and these theories are further explored in subsequent chapters.

Throughout this chapter, it has become clear that a symbiotic relationship has developed between the medical profession and the state, a relationship of mutual dependence. But debate about health policy continues to be carried out in the shadow of a complex web of mutual dependencies between government and the profession which support a 'shifting assembly of pacts and bargains, both formally negotiated and tacitly understood' (Harrison et al. 1990: 2). This has had many positive side-effects. It has

meant that each side remains sensitive to the needs of the other and that successive ministers have placed emphasis on consulting with those who contribute so much to the service being provided. To do otherwise would surely bring with it the risk of sterile policies. But it has also meant that the profession's constant vigilance over its jurisdiction and what remains politically acceptable makes it more likely that changes will tend to come from within the profession. Even the DoH's recently published consultation document on the reform of the GMC was developed *by* the GMC. Such moves could be seen to represent greater efforts to retain control, through internal agreement, by forestalling the need for external intervention in the GMC's work. Paradoxically, while these measures may reduce the individual clinician's autonomy, they also signal a movement towards greater rather than lesser conformity to the ideal type of self-regulating professional group. In the next chapter these general political shifts will be discussed and explained by reference to specific policy developments relating to complaints.

Notes

1 Interestingly, commentators on the politics of the NHS have come up with some notable exceptions to this approach during the birth and growth of a nationalized health service in the UK. Cartwright (1977) has described in his book on the creation of the NHS how Lloyd-George introduced the National Health Insurance Bill in 1911 without prior discussion of its contents with the medical profession. Cartwright contends that it was only in the course of negotiations about how it would be implemented that the BMA began to appreciate that it involved new bureaucratic controls over doctors. Klein (1989) gives the example of Bevan's handling of the debate about the setting up of the NHS, which was much more open than was usual.

2 Although Oxford University offered courses in medicine from the early thirteenth century, training as a physician remained a largely intellectual endeavour and more time was spent studying arts subjects than the body and its ailments. While being a physician was considered to be a gentlemanly pursuit during this period and for many years to come, those who acted as barber surgeons and grocer apothecaries were considered to be artisans conducting a trade. The first Medical Act was enacted in 1511 as a result of Henry VIII's concerns about the lack of skill and education exhibited by many practitioners. The Act made it an offence for anyone to practise medicine or surgery unless they were a graduate of a university or had been licensed by a bishop after examination, but did little to enforce proper training. Despite the considerable overlap in the type of work undertaken by physicians and apothecaries it was not until the 1815 Apothecaries Act that legislation

governing the latter's educational qualification was passed. The 1815 Act empowered the Society of Apothecaries to prosecute throughout England those who practised medicine without having undertaken the right education and training. Interestingly, the scope of powers allowed by the 1815 Act was broader than those in earlier legislation. In the case of physicians and barber surgeons their power to oversee the work of colleagues was limited to controlling practice within London and ensuring the purity of drugs issued by apothecaries.

3   This was the first time that physicians, surgeons and apothecaries had argued for joint recognition.

4   During this time, a number of groups, such as those representing physicians', surgeons' and apothecaries' associations, struggled to occupy a position of superior status to others (MacDonald 1995). Some contemporary critics objected strongly to the setting up of the monopolistic GMC because it was thought to offend the dominant ideology of *laissez-faire*. Its establishment was perceived as a threat to an unregulated market and it took a number of parliamentary debates and Bills before politicians were convinced that the move towards a monopoly was in the public interest. Even then, it may be that it was pragmatism rather than principle which eventually provided a convincing reason for the introduction of a single licensing agency. Cartwright (1977) has argued that it was the practical need of government to have a simple register to appoint medical officers of health during a series of epidemics in the mid-nineteenth century which was, in the end, the greatest force for change.

5   Twenty licensing bodies continued to operate after the Act was in force but their activities were overseen by the GMC. The Act did not impose a single qualification as there was too much disagreement on the issue from factions within the profession.

6   It was largely during this time that doctors came to dominate the emerging hospital sector.

7   In her discussion of this crucial period, Allsop (1995) describes how there continued to be a division of interests between hospital doctors, GPs, politicians, public health specialists in local authorities and the voluntary sector. She claims that this was resolved by compromise on all fronts but that hospital consultants did particularly well out of the resulting deal (see also Gill 1971). Hospital doctors were given the right to continue with their private practice alongside their new NHS work, able to maintain a high degree of control over conditions of appointment and granted control over a new merit award system set up to reward high achievers. Significantly, teaching hospitals staffed by the elite of the profession were given special status (Ham 1992) and medics were also able to negotiate considerable control over expenditure and the development of policies in hospitals. In short, there was a trade-off of interests. The public ownership of hospitals suited the Labour

government of the day and the steady flow of regular income suited hospital doctors.

8   At the time that preliminary discussions were taking place there were two sorts of hospital in existence – the municipal hospitals, which were under local authority control, and the voluntary hospitals where most doctors undertook their training. It had become clear in the 1920s that the voluntary hospitals were experiencing a serious financial crisis.

9   The profession was particularly disturbed by the argument made in the Brown Plan of 1943 that doctors working for the NHS should become full-time salaried staff. Brown was the Minister for Health in 1942 but is reported to have given up the job shortly afterwards because of his frustration at being unable to achieve consensus within and without the profession.

10   This was a plan put forward in the Brown Plan (1943) and was repeated in Henry Willink's White Paper of 1944.

11   The notion of local government control was scrapped and the administration of municipal hospitals was transferred from local government centres to new regional authorities and new hospital boards.

12   The medical profession was particularly successful in getting agreement that doctors should not be salaried employees and could work part-time and carry out private work in addition to their contract with the NHS.

13   The claims of doctors to these concessions were undoubtedly aided in debate by the fact that the subservience of workers in this plan did not accord with one of the primary objects in the Labour Party manifesto which was a greater partnership with the worker in the management of their trade (Cartwright 1977).

14   In other areas the profession was not so successful. It is particularly noticeable that some groups of doctors fared less well than others in the negotiation process. Secondary care was privileged at the expense of primary care which, in turn, attracted more resources than public health.

15   The granting of study leave, travel expenses and special merit awards to hospital consultants are a testament to this.

16   These local executive councils also oversaw the work of pharmaceutical, ophthalmic and dental services.

17   See also the CHI investigation of lung and heart transplantation at St George's NHS Trust, the employment of locums and the removal of the wrong kidney at Carmarthenshire NHS Trust, the CHI's clinical governance reports on the Mid-Cheshire Hospital NHS Trust, Ipswich Hospital NHS Trust, Pinderfields and Pontefract NHS Hospitals Trust and Rotherham General Hospitals Trust.

18   Klein (1989) cites the battle over the presence of private beds in NHS hospitals spearheaded by Barbara Castle as an example of socialists calling in an overdue debt to the Labour Party's socialist ideals.

19 Prior to the Griffiths Report in 1983 (DHSS 1983b) the NHS was run by consensus teams with doctors and nurses sharing responsibilities with administrators for spending. Attempts to get doctors to help manage the service were made but were largely unsuccessful (see, e.g. Ministry of Health 1967). Reforms introduced in the wake of the Griffiths Report turned administrators into general managers who had overall responsibility for budgetary control of health care. Post-Griffiths, medical representatives on management teams lost their veto power and general managers were introduced at all levels of the NHS machinery. Significantly, managers had a direct interest in the promotion of change because their salaries were directly linked to performance.

20 Initiatives launched in the wake of the *Working for Patients* White Paper required that all consultants should have job descriptions which included details of how much time they spent on NHS work.

21 However, evidence about the willingness of doctors to participate in hospital-wide risk management and audit structures suggests that, despite these moves, a culture of resistance to managerial authority continues to exist (Berwick et al. 1992a, 1992b; Allsop and Mulcahy 1996). Research suggests that, in practice, managers have made only limited inroads into professional autonomy (Flynn 1991). Despite their reliance on scientific models in their claims for legitimacy, Harper Mills and Bolschwing (1995) suggest that doctors have not embraced calls for the collection of data about their own clinical conduct. Reporting on their experience in US hospitals, they comment, for instance, that doctors became protective when their own information was being screened for quality analysis.

22 Trusts can seek the advice of the NCAA at an early stage where a doctor appears to be failing. The NCAA may work with a doctor or Trust to identify problems with organizational structure or training and development needs. The aim of the NCAA is to complement and support the work of employers and the GMC in addressing the professional performance of individual practitioners (DoH 2002).

23 These developments are discussed more widely in Chapter 5, on the complainant's perspective, as they provide an important context for a fuller understanding of complaints as a form of protest.

24 The position was summarized in 1978 by the Normansfield Report:

> At the inception of the NHS, the Government made clear that its intention was to provide a framework within which the health profession could provide treatment and care for patients according to their own independent professional judgement of the patient's needs. Their independence has continued to be a central feature of the organization and management of health services. Thus, hospital consultants have clinical autonomy and are fully responsible for the treatment they prescribe

for their patients. They are required to act within broad limits of acceptable medical practice and within policy for the use of resources, but they are not held accountable to NHS authorities for their clinical judgements.

(DHSS 1978a: 424–5)

3 An inspector calls
The emergence of complaints procedures

Introduction

This chapter aims to expose the various ways in which the elite of the profession have attempted to insulate doctors from managerial intervention in complaints handling and maintained the professional model of regulation. Tracing the development of NHS complaints procedures provides a useful study of how the professional project discussed in the previous chapter came to be achieved and how considerable powers continue to be reserved for doctors at service level to self-manage complaints about their work. The design and reform of complaints procedures within the NHS have been hotly contested. Professional bodies have lobbied hard to retain control over the initial stages of all complaint handling, and over all stages of clinical complaint handling. By reviewing the policy negotiations which have taken place behind the formal regulations governing complaints, I have attempted to reveal both the underbelly of political debate and the ways in which the macro-level debates about professional power discussed in the previous chapter have come to manifest themselves in discussions of complaints.

It is argued that the profession's claim to autonomy and self-regulation has been a successful one. Despite shifts in debate towards a consumer-oriented model and rights discourse, doctors continue to have considerable discretion over complaint handling at service level. Increasing emphasis has been placed on the procedural fairness of appeals procedures so that the arguments of complainant and doctor are given equal weight, but there is little regulation of front-line handling of complaints and guidance on the circumstances in which complaints should be referred further up the hierarchy is vague. For doctors, the new arrangements for complaint handling introduced in 1996 appear to have considerable benefits. They now have the opportunity for early notification of dissatisfaction and time to resolve an issue before it escalates. But the procedures do little to enhance the power of the service user who is still in the weaker position of being at the receiving end of a largely monopolistic service. Neither do present procedures enhance the powers of the state in its attempt to ensure fair and consistent handling of citizen grievances. Instead they reveal a tension between the needs of a number of actors – individual complainants, providers of medical services, the general public and the state in regulating medical work. Regulation of powerful groups in society has always been something of a daunting task for the state and one which has been boldly attempted as part of the shift towards marketization of the public sector. But in its attempts to encourage informalism and responsiveness, in the consumer interest, the NHS Executive may have got the balance between these competing interests wrong and provided insufficient checks on the handling of grievances.

Early attempts at managing complaints

It can be assumed that complaints about the quality of care have been a feature of medical work since the time when medical assistance was first given. But, until the mid-nineteenth century, there appears to have been no public debate about the need for an integrated approach to complaint handling. Until that period, the state had a minimal role in the regulation of medical work and played a much less interventionist role in society than the modern state. Framing responses to complaints was a matter for the individual practitioner and their conscience. This situation changed when the GMC was set up by the Medical Act of 1858. Handling complaints about poor practice which might warrant deregistration was identified as a core function of the GMC and constituted a key part of the bargain struck with the state at its inception (Stacey 1992). At the time it followed naturally from the granting of monopoly power to the GMC over who should be allowed to enter the profession, that they should also be expected to determine who should be expelled. The contemporary choice was viewed as being between a self-regulated market for medical care and an unregulated one (Allsop 1998).

Thus, in return for being given competitive advantage in the market, doctors recognized by the GMC were required to stabilize the profession's internal institutional arrangements through the GMC (Belant 1975). This resulted in the introduction of a mechanism for the expulsion of doctors found guilty of serious professional misconduct. The standard was a minimal one but has only very recently been changed. Critics have suggested that the high threshold of incompetence originally put in place as the criterion for expulsion has meant that in reality the vast majority of doctors complained about to the GMC have had the case against them dismissed (Smith 1994). But, at the time the GMC was being established, it was conceded that as long as it made an effort to discipline poorly performing doctors then the state would respect its claim to clinical autonomy and allow self-regulation. For well over a century after the GMC was established, formal complaints were limited to these atypical cases.

Complaint handling systems operating outside the one overseen by the GMC have been slow to follow. Even when the NHS was created in 1948 the state declined to take responsibility for overseeing or managing complaint handling by doctors. Stacey (1992) has explained that policy makers initially thought to enforce the same model of accountability for doctors which applied to bureaucrats within the NHS. This had a certain logic as both administrators and doctors were employees of the NHS. But it was successfully argued by the profession that the nature of medicine was such that purpose-designed arrangements would be needed which would run in parallel with bureaucratic models. The tension between the bureaucratic and self-regulatory models reflected an aversion on the part of doctors to being line-managed by bureaucrats or other doctors and concern lest the special nature of medical work went unrecognized.[1] As a result, when the NHS came into being doctors inherited dual responsibilities: to their employers[2] and to the GMC. Although the Health Service Commissioner's (HSC) post was created by the legislature in 1973,[3] the remit of the role was restricted for over 20 years to non-clinical complaints. Moreover, it was only in the latter half of the twentieth century that the common law properly recognized the right of patients to sue doctors for medical negligence (Mason and McCall-Smith 1994). Despite this, there remains much evidence to suggest that the courts have avoided imposing exacting standards on doctors.

The specific focus of this book is on hospital complaints procedures but it is relevant to note that a highly restricted and minimal complaints system developed in the primary care sector at the inception of the NHS. Since 1946 health authorities with responsibility for overseeing the primary care sector have made contracts with self-employed medics to provide general practitioner services. Doctors who agreed to be placed on the local lists of qualified practitioners prepared to act as general practitioners agreed to be bound by nationally negotiated terms of service which outlined their responsibilities. Patients or relatives who were dissatisfied with the service provided could complain to the local health authority* to have their grievance heard by a local Medical Service Committee (MSC). These bodies actually had their origin in the 1911 Insurance Act but various NHS regulations have, over the years governed their operation.

MSCs acted as judicial style tribunals, were subject to the supervisory jurisdiction of the Council on Tribunals and used the Bolam test as the standard of care. The terms of service which formed the basis of the MSC's terms of reference run to hundreds of pages but most cases centred on two paragraphs

---

* Initially these were called Executive Councils, then Family Practitioner Committees and later Family Health Service Authorities.

which related to doctors' duties to attend patients out of hours and their discretion to refer patients to hospitals. These very specific issues which formed the core of the responsibilities over which practitioners could be held to account and the limitations of the Bolam principle meant that, in effect, the jurisdiction of these tribunals was extremely limited and that many dissatisfied patients had no jurisdiction to use the procedure. Apart from the personal satisfaction at bringing poor performance to light, a patient also received little direct benefit from pursuing their complaint in this way. Service committees were, and continue to be, empowered to give a warning, withhold a sum of money from the doctor's remuneration, request that the doctor pay the complainant's expenses or recommend that their name be struck off the local list.

Within the hospital sector regional hospital boards, boards of governors and hospital management committees dealt with complaints about hospital services without any detailed advice from the government other than that relating to serious disciplinary matters for the first two decades of the NHS (DHSS 1973). Until 1966, complaints procedures in the hospital sector were largely unstructured and varied between hospitals and districts. Centralized guidance from the Department of Health and Social Security (DHSS) was circulated that year but tended to concentrate on atypical complaint handling scenarios involving the setting up of occasional independent *ad hoc* committees to investigate the most serious complaints, such as physical abuse of patients by hospital staff.

It was not until 20 years after the creation of the NHS that an attempt was made at standardization of local complaint handling practices within hospitals with the circulation of *Health Memorandum (HM(66)15)* (DHSS 1966). This brief, 850-word document privileged medical discourse above others. It recommended the adoption of skeletal procedures in which much discretion to set up a complaints procedure was left to those providing the care being criticized. Three particular features of the 1966 guidance are worthy of note and each of them reflects a preference for local and informal self-regulation by the profession. First, it allowed for handling of complaints about doctors to be conducted almost exclusively by doctors. Second, there was little opportunity for grievances to be considered by others outside the organization involved in the complaint. This situation was exacerbated by ambiguity about how and to what extent members of hospital authorities should be involved with, or informed about, investigations of complaints. Finally, the memorandum was not binding on hospitals or clinicians. Instead, it was anticipated that local providers would complement its broad statements of principle with detailed rules at service level.

The memorandum recommended that all complaints should be dealt with promptly and complainants made aware that their complaints had been fully and fairly considered. In addition, the memorandum recommended a crude appeals procedure. This left considerable discretion in the hands of practitioners at service level as to how appeals should be managed. The guidance advised that oral complaints which could not be dealt with to the complainant's satisfaction should be reported to a senior member of staff in the same department, who should make a brief note of the complaint and take 'appropriate' action. In cases where the complainant wanted to take the matter beyond this level it was recommended that a written complaint be directed to the hospital management committee or a senior member of staff. Action taken in response to the complaint was to be agreed, after consultation, with the head of department concerned. It was only complaints that could not be dealt with satisfactorily in this way that had to be reported to the hospital management committee or to 'an appropriate committee' for a decision as to further action. Where this was considered necessary the case could be referred to the Regional Hospital Board which was empowered to establish an inquiry chaired by an independent lawyer.

By the mid-1970s a series of government inquiries into poor quality in hospitals provided an extraordinary environment in which more radical inroads into clinical autonomy during complaint handling could be contemplated. When the Ely (DHSS 1969), Fairleigh (DHSS 1971), Whittingham (DHSS 1972) and Normansfield (DHSS 1978a) Inquiries reported, they highlighted the need for a thorough review of hospital complaints procedures. More strategically, they hinted at serious failure in the regulatory compact between the profession and the state which had been made at the time the GMC was established. The inquiries made serious allegations about neglect of vulnerable patient groups, such as elderly people and those with learning disadvantages. The deficiencies highlighted related to nursing and medical standards, facilities and custodial attitudes towards care (Ham 1992). Significantly, the inquiries were partly set up as a consequence of the failure of internal NHS complaints procedures to highlight quality issues and pointed to the need for more effective monitoring of hospital services (Crossman 1972; DHSS 1973). Public outrage ensued on the publication of the reports and criticisms of doctors focused on the suppression of complaints and the victimization of staff who complained on behalf of patients. Hospital management committees were also shown to have failed to provide safeguards or remedies for such abuses. The Ely Hospital inquiry in particular encouraged the issues raised to become generalized into a wider concern about social justice and humanitarian values. As a result of the publicity, pressure group activity and ministerial concern, the DHSS set about reviewing the reasons for the failure of complaints procedures to identify poor practice. Soon after the publication of the reports, the Hospital Advisory Service was set up to improve and oversee the management of long-stay hospitals and the possibility of introducing an HSC was widely debated. Moreover, within a few years of the abuses coming to light, the DHSS also set up a committee under the chairmanship of Sir Michael Davies to look more generally at the problems with hospital complaints procedures. Stacey (1999) has argued that doctors gave their support to this initiative because they feared that, unless complaints were adequately handled, there would be an escalation of medical negligence claims in the aftermath of public discussions of the scandals.

The Davies Committee on hospital complaints

The Davies Committee was the first government-sanctioned investigation of the NHS hospital complaints procedure.[4] Its Report (DHSS 1973) remains the most comprehensive and in-depth review of its kind to have been undertaken in the UK.[5] Much of the discussion contained in it remains relevant to contemporary debates about complaint procedures and reflects tensions among providers of services which are still prevalent today. It is significant that the chair of the Committee was a high-court judge, and the investigatory style he adopted was formal, legalistic and evidence-based. As a result, the duties of NHS employees and government departments were discussed in the context of formal responsibilities and channels of authority. The Report provides a stark contrast with the Wilson Committee review of NHS complaints procedures, conducted exactly 20 years later, under the chairmanship of a university vice chancellor, Alan Wilson, which was asked to report in four months and appears to have been influenced much less by the formal evidence submitted to it (Stacey and Moss 1996).[6] The Davies Committee undertook its own empirical research,[7] met formally on 30 occasions, held several other informal sessions and invited written evidence.[8]

The Committee had four major criticisms of the 1966 procedure which were subsequently to become familiar themes in reviews of NHS complaints procedures. Each suggested a failure on the part of practitioners to take complaints seriously. It found defensive attitudes to complaints were common and appeared to be having a detrimental effect on staff morale. This encouraged indifference to complaint handling and tended to repress grievances. In addition, inadequate information was available to staff and complainants about complaints procedures and how they might be accessed, and there was no effective system of external checks in operation on how well complaints were being managed. Finally, the Committee felt that inadequate attention was being paid to encouraging complaints, most of which were thought to be but a small challenge to medicine or its administration. Research commissioned by the Committee supported the view that hospital staff had operated the procedures in a way which insulated them from criticism. It was found that there was an unwillingness to activate the 'appeals' procedure with the result that those determined to pursue their case were encouraged to turn to the courts.[9] In addition, the challenge of supplementing the rather vague procedure outlined in the governing memorandum by the introduction of a more detailed local one had not been taken up by local providers of NHS services.

Significantly, the Report also revealed that, under the 1966 procedure, consultants maintained considerable control over the everyday investigation of both clinical and non-clinical complaints. In a survey of all 330 hospital boards operating in England and Wales, it was found that three main categories of postholder were responsible for the investigation of complaints which could not be dealt with adequately at service level. These were group secretaries, hospital secretaries (administrators) and professionals or heads of departments.[10] While professionals had little *formal responsibility* for complaint handling (8 per cent of those who responded to the survey were responsible for complaints about standards in patient care), an entirely different picture emerges from survey data on who actually *conducted* investigations and suggests that doctors wielded considerable power over the process. Professionals or heads of department were responsible for conducting 70 per cent (291) of investigations about medical treatment; 73 per cent (284) of cases about treatment facilities; and 82 per cent (291) of complaints about the standard of care. These data raised important issues about the effectiveness of self-regulation as the Committee identified concerns that doctors who handled complaints were more likely than others to adopt a reactive approach to them. Consultants were seen by colleagues and patient groups as particularly unwilling to review or evaluate the clinical judgement of another hospital consultant and jeopardize a fellow doctor's reputation, especially where litigation might be involved. Many were not prepared to become involved in investigations at all and, in any case, fear of litigation often inhibited full investigation.

Recommendations made by the Committee

The Davies Report was published in 1973. Where the 1966 guidance was vague and opaque, the 82 recommendations made by the Davies Committee were complex and intricate. The Report argued that existing guidance on complaints was too narrow and an insufficient aid to practice, concentrating as it did on broad principles and the responsibilities of those at higher managerial levels. It identified a number of principles which should steer the design of complaint procedures but also drafted more specific guidance on how such procedures should operate on a day-to-day basis. It recommended that complaints must be properly investigated, a fair review or evaluation of the allegation made, and remedial action taken or a reasoned explanation given as to why this was not appropriate. Significantly, the Committee was strongly of the view that external involvement in complaint handling was essential. It designed a somewhat convoluted new complaints procedure for hospitals, with tangential procedures being established where a clear course of action could not be decided upon. At its simplest, it allowed for a four-stage procedure which would involve increasing amounts of external involvement as complaints progressed through it. The Committee anticipated that doctors would be particularly critical of these proposals but concluded that fair and visible procedures were essential:

> This improvement is in the interests of complainants, who have a right to expect that their complaints will be fully and impartially considered; in the interests of professional staff, whose action may have been misrepresented or misunderstood; and in the interests of good management by health authorities, who are responsible for administering administrative defects or failures of service that may not otherwise be brought to light.
>
> (DHSS 1973: 65)

In this way, the Committee shifted the focus of concern away from notions of how the public good could be determined by practitioners, towards a discourse of individual rights. Unlike previous guidance, it stressed not only the responsibilities of health providers but the *rights* of patients. Complaining was characterized as a legitimate activity and public bodies were presented as having particular responsibilities to those they treated. In support of this approach it was argued that 'a public body is under a higher duty to disclose matters which have gone wrong ... It should proceed on the basis that it is more important to investigate complaints and put matters right that have gone wrong than simply to protect itself' (DHSS 1973: 78).

Moreover, the Committee made clear that, as far as accountability was concerned, doctors did not enjoy a special status. It was argued that the duties which public servants owed to service users applied equally to administrators and professionals:

> We believe that people who complain about medical treatment should never be given the reply that the complaint (or part of it) cannot be investigated 'because it involves the exercise of clinical judgement'. They are entitled to a full answer from the consultant concerned and the hospital authority in our view has a clear duty to make sure they get it.
>
> (DHSS 1973: 44)

Moreover, unlike official commentaries which preceded or postdated its investigation, the Davies Report recognized the potential conflict between clinicians and manager-bureaucrats when managing complaints by anticipating that consultants and managers might well disagree about how complaints should be responded to.[11]

But, while the language of consumerism, procedural fairness and managerial responsibility for complaint handling is rife within the Davies Report, its most significant recommendations did much to further the cause of those committed to clinical autonomy and self-regulation. The Report set important precedents which have subsequently served to insulate the profession from external regulation of complaints. Despite evidence that doctors were reluctant to criticize each other and that the profession was not fulfilling its side of its regulatory pact with the state, the Davies Committee differentiated between the handling of complaints about the exercise of clinical judgement and other complaints. Its membership was persuaded of the apparent necessity of this approach by evidence about the distinctiveness and complexity of clinical complaints submitted by the profession. Upon what information was such an assumption based? Thirty per cent of hospital authorities who responded to the Committee's survey identified clinical complaints as the most difficult to handle and resolve, followed by only 14 per cent of hospital authorities who believed that complaints about the attitude of staff were the most problematic. Clinical complaints were perceived as different because the task of establishing the validity of a complaint was more complex. In the words of one hospital authority cited in the Report:

> Obviously [complaints] with medical overtones tend to be more difficult than those allied to nursing and lay administration. With the clinical freedom enjoyed by medical staff the method of treatment and approach differs between doctors and, what may be acceptable to one patient or to one doctor is looked upon with disfavour by another patient or another doctor.
>
> (DHSS 1973: 18)

The commentary emphasizes two key factors which have been used to distinguish professional from lay work – the emphasis on specialized knowledge and the emphasis on the *art* of practising medicine. Read carefully, the quotation admits of the possibility that no medical work can be criticized. By accepting the distinction between clinical and non-clinical complaints, the Committee acceded to the claim of the profession to regulate challenges to the medical fraternity. Accordingly, it recommended that complaints about medical care should, in the first instance, be dealt with by the doctor responsible for the medical care being criticized. Where they could not be resolved informally in this way, it was suggested that they should be referred to another medical consultant and that consultant was expected to agree a response with a chief officer of the hospital authority. Only after that could dissatisfied complainants refer the complaint to an independent investigating panel. These rationales for separating clinical and non-clinical complaints have proved influential and remained virtually unquestioned until recent years.

On reflection, it is clear that the Davies Committee made an important contribution to the debate about the handling of complaints. It recognized many of the problems which deterred patients and their carers from voicing grievances and the serious consequences of inadequate procedures when provision of care went seriously wrong. The Committee expressed its commitment to the right to complain and get an adequate response. It also supported the managerial coordination of complaints and the importance of using legally qualified chairs in appeal mechanisms. In supporting such initiatives it hoped to introduce a legal-bureaucratic structure underpinned by notions of due process to a predominantly medical model. It even suggested that these factors would challenge medical determinations of responsibility by subjecting them to opinions and suggestions which came from outside the professional group. Perhaps most importantly the Committee suggested a design for the complaints procedure which paid heed to some of the principles of procedural justice. In these ways it placed primary emphasis on the mechanics of accountability to the public rather than just to the professional group.

But the rhetoric of accountability was not applied with such vigour to complaints about clinical care as it was to other complaints. The same barrier was inserted between the medical and administrative sphere as had characterized the organization of the NHS since its inception. This achievement is all the more remarkable because it occurred at a time of extraordinary negotiation between the state and the profession, in which there were important prizes to be fought for and won in the contemporary discussion of how the NHS should be organized. As Margaret Stacey, a member of the Davies Committee, later reflected:

> the doctors worked hard to have the machinery the way they wanted it: for example, a veto was put on recommendations that a notice about the complaints procedure should be widely displayed in wards, out-patients departments and so on. We were told that would damage the doctor-patient relationship which was painted as sacred. A patrician attitude was much in evidence.
>
> (Stacey 1999: 2)

Support for the Committee's recommendations was not universal. In a private interview, Stacey (1999) has explained how a minority of Committee members, including herself and a senior medic, considered submitting a minority report to the DHSS because of their concern about the level of compromise agreed with the profession. The group was dissuaded from doing so by Sir Michael Davies himself and the disgruntled members were swayed by the impending announcements about the introduction of a Health Service Ombudsman. But, in time, they were to become disenchanted about the 'thundering silence' which followed the Report and Michael Davies' 'unwillingness to stir it' (Stacey 1999). The Report was not even referred to in any of the official guidance, executive letters or circulars which came after it. Margaret Stacey later reflected that the compromise reached was unattractive to all stakeholders:

> At this stage, I became sorry I had agreed a compromise at a last minute breakfast meeting. A radical minority report might have attracted more attention to the complaints debate and the Davies report. After about 10 years, a complaints system emerged, but what a mouse it was. I learned later from an authoritative source that the Royal College of Physicians had held progress up and had relegated a member of the College who had been on the Davies Committee to a backwater for signing the report.
>
> (Stacey 1999: 3)

As Stacey suggested, the recommendations of the Davies Committee were not immediately translated into new guidance. The handling of clinical complaints does not appear to have been the subject of further review until it was considered by the DHSS in the light of an independent review of the subject by a House of Commons Select Committee in 1977. This report brought fresh regulatory challenges to the profession. In its first and subsequent reports, the Select Committee emphasized the need for appeal structures as well as front-line handling of complaints by doctors. It recommended that the independent appraisal of complaints should be the task of a lay HSC, and that the HSC should be given the scope to review the operation of the handling of clinical complaints and any complaints which health authorities could not resolve (Select Committee 1977–8).

As a result of the pressures exerted by the Select Committee and repeated fears about increasing litigation, the Joint Consultants' Committee (JCC) of the BMA and Royal Colleges produced its own set of recommendations on how clinical complaints should be handled. These reflected a more overt attempt at maintaining control over clinical complaint handling than had previously been the case and rested on the assumption that the distinction between clinical and non-clinical complaints should be maintained. They suggested that while complaints about organizational or administrative aspects of medical care and treatment should be investigated by health authorities, complaints concerning clinical judgement should be handled by clinicians. Even the principle that there should be an independent review of clinical complaints was not accepted. The notion of review was not rejected but it was argued that, where complainants were not satisfied with the handling of clinical complaints at service level, these could be referred to a panel of two senior clinicians for further consideration. The recommendations were not without their attractions to consumer groups. The stated aim of such a review panel was to provide a less formal redress procedure than that provided by the courts. It was argued that complainants who sought an investigation and an explanation of their case, rather than punitive measures or compensation, should have somewhere to take their concerns in order to have them addressed (Watson 1992). But, the recommendations were described by the Association of Community Health Councils in England and Wales (ACHCEW) (1990) as a deliberate attempt to forestall other attempts at closer regulation of doctors' work and, in particular, to resist the otherwise likely extension of the Ombudsman's role to include clinical complaint handling. Others have described them as a simple 'fudge' (Stacey 1992).

The emergence of a separate clinical complaints procedure

The DHSS issued a substantial draft code of practice for complaint handling and circulated it for comment in June 1976 (DHSS 1976). Significantly, the protocol accepted the distinction between clinical and non-clinical complaints, but it did this by concentrating on non-clinical complaints and avoiding the issue of how clinical complaints should be managed. The draft code reflected many of the concerns of the Davies Committee. In particular it suggested that complaints procedures should be publicized; complainants should be assisted in making complaints; complaints should be recorded; and that they should be referred to a more senior level if necessary. But while the principle of managerial control of complaint handling was accepted in relation to the handling of non-clinical complaints, this was not the case where complaints involving clinical judgement were concerned. Appendix 4 of the document reproduced the guidelines drafted by the JCC for the separate handling of clinical complaints and in this way the foundations were laid for a parallel system for clinical complaints which was to last two decades.

The draft code was followed in 1978 with a further consultation document, *Health Note (HN(78)39)* (DHSS 1978b), which took account of the comments of health authorities and other interested parties. It claimed to reflect the 'widespread' (p. 1) view that the arrangements proposed were too detailed and complex and that a simple procedure was needed. This recommendation was in direct contrast to that made by the Davies Committee which had felt that much tighter regulation of complaint handling was necessary. As was the case with the draft code of 1976, this consultation document did not deal with the handling of clinical complaints as this issue was still being considered separately in light of the Select Committee's first report. However, it was followed in 1981 by *Health Circular (HC(81)5)* (DHSS 1981) on the subject. Despite the lack of full or public consultation on the clinical complaints procedure, the Circular incorporated the trial procedure suggested by the draft code of practice in 1976 and made clear that this had been formally agreed between the DHSS and the JCC. It is significant that while non-clinical complaints were considered worthy of full consultation with interested stakeholders, arrangements for the handling of clinical complaints were negotiated between the profession and the DHSS in a more private and less visible forum.

The medical profession worked hard to persuade policy makers that the new trial procedure was a success. In 1983 the DHSS circulated a brief report on the operation of the third stage of the new procedure which involved an Independent Professional Review (IPR) of the kind originally suggested by the BMA and Royal Colleges. The report drew on data supplied by doctors and NHS managers (DHSS 1983a) and concluded that, on the basis of this, the new trial 'appeals' procedure had been a success, although the views of complainants and patient groups were not sought. In support of this contention, it was reported that the independent assessors appointed to review the work of colleagues had received the full cooperation of the doctors involved and had gained access to the health records of patients in all cases. In government circles the new procedures were praised as satisfying the compact between the state and the profession. Shortly after the report was published, the then Minister for Health, Kenneth Clarke argued:

> The procedure is still at an early stage, and we will continue to watch progress to see whether we have effectively provided patients and relatives with the response to complaints to which they are entitled. But it is already clear that the medical profession has responded constructively. 'Second opinions' have given frank and expert assessments, and their colleagues whose actions they have scrutinised have offered full co-operation.
>
> (DHSS 1983a: 2)

Despite such assertions, the DHSS report also revealed that decision making during the reviews was dominated by medical opinion including that of the doctor complained about. It demonstrated that, on receipt of a referral, the regional medical officers charged with the discretion of calling for an IPR asked for and studied all relevant case notes and correspondence. But, while they discussed the matter with medical staff involved, they rarely chose to visit the complainant as part of their review.

Further changes to the hospital complaints procedure were prompted, quite fortuitously by the chance intervention of a back-bench MP in 1985 who argued for reform from an entirely different perspective. His interest in improving communication and accountability for health service users led to his private member's bill getting the backing of government and becoming law. In a private interview with the author, Sir Michael McNair Wilson, he described to me how the impetus for reform came about when he was hospital-

ized for a kidney complaint and became concerned about the lack of information available to patients. His response was to draft a patient's charter which
placed emphasis on the service user's needs rather than on those of professionals. When he secured a place in the private members' ballot, he decided
to try and transform his charter into legislation but the Secretary of State for
Health informed him that this initiative would not get government backing
unless he chose just one clause of the charter to form a Bill. He selected the
clause relating to hospital complaints and his Bill became law in 1985 as the
Hospital Complaint (Procedure) Act. This continues to be the only piece of primary legislation governing the operation of the hospital complaints procedure
(McNair-Wilson 1989).

This legislation made it compulsory for the first time that all hospitals put
in place a procedure for complaint handling. In promoting the Bill, which
received all-party backing, Sir Michael emphasized the needs of patients over
those of doctors. In parliamentary debate he posed the questions:

> Whose chance? Whose life? Whose body? Who is the sufferer? What
> is the compensation? What is the complaints procedure? There
> appears to be no such procedure. The patient is just the fall guy who is
> in the hands of doctors who think they know better than the patient.
> (McNair-Wilson 1989)

The Act was well received across the political spectrum. Lord Winstanley
described Lord Colwyn's introduction of the Bill in the House of Lords as
being in a mood of 'benevolent neutrality'.[12] Ministers are reported to have
welcomed the opportunity the Bill provided for the re-examination of existing
complaints procedures and for ensuring that the procedure commanded the
confidence of the public, health authorities and health professionals alike. But
despite such laudable aims, the legislation was described elsewhere as 'modest'
(Brazier 1987: 126). With only two sections, the second of which constitutes
the short title, it is only notable because it forced health authorities to set up a
formal complaints procedure in compliance with centrally agreed guidelines.
The guidelines themselves were still left to be negotiated with the profession.
In fact, it took three years for guidance to be issued under the Act (DHSS 1988).
When guidance did appear, it served to rubber-stamp the arrangements made
between the DHSS and JCC in 1976. The dual systems for handling clinical and
non-clinical complaints were justified by the Minister for Health and Social
Security who suggested that the ideal of self-regulation alone was appropriate
to place boundaries on clinical autonomy. Apparently, unaware of the precedent set by the establishment of the GMC in 1858, he described the procedure
as an 'important innovation, because doctors have now accepted responsibility for scrutinizing and assessing the clinical actions of colleagues' (DHSS
1983b: 10).

It was not until a decade later that there was some discussion in policy circles about the need to update the complaints procedure in the light of reforms to the NHS and the patient's charter initiative. Supporters of the status quo remained sensitive to the need to persuade other stakeholders of the value of a bifurcated system. In 1992, when the IPR had been in operation for ten years, the JCC seized the opportunity to conduct its own review of the procedure which drew on reports to the JCC from independent clinical assessors who had adjudicated appeals. It concluded that the procedure had an important role in monitoring and improving patient satisfaction and that, in the majority of cases, it was of value to the complainant and doctor involved.

The review also reported some concerns about the threat of independent regulation of medical work by the HSC and an increase in the web of controls. The JCC was concerned that the HSC had been reviewing cases which had gone to an IPR and worried that consultants would be less likely to act as assessors if they thought their actions would be subject to review.[13] It was also argued that the HSC's intervention had served to change the interpretation of the guidance which the JCC had negotiated with the DoH. At the time the HSC was specifically precluded from investigating complaints relating to actions taken solely in consequence of clinical judgement but he considered it within his jurisdiction to review regional medical officer decisions on whether an IPR should be held. This meant that the HSC could force an IPR to be held if necessary. Such intervention clearly sought to blur the distinctions traditionally drawn between the clinical and non-clinical procedures. The threat was much more than an academic one about boundaries. It was about this time that the HSC began to make public his view that his office was capable of overseeing clinical and non-clinical complaint handling. The views of such a high-ranking lawyer were somewhat harder to undermine than those made by patient groups and served to fuel other criticisms of the procedure throughout the late 1980s and early 1990s.

Growing concern about complaint handling

During this same period, criticisms that the hospital complaints procedure tended to protect the interests of doctors over those of patients were widespread among the HSC, patient and complainant advocates, the Select Committee and academics. Concerns were expressed that the clinical complaints procedure was too complex, attracted insufficient publicity and that responses to patients were poor and defensive. In the words of one critic speaking on behalf of Community Health Councils (CHCs):

> The processes for airing grievances, investigating complaints and providing explanations when things go wrong are considered by

those who use them to be long winded, cumbersome, bureaucratic and strongly weighted in favour of the medical profession.

(ACHCEW 1990: 15)[14]

The Patients Association claimed that the clinical complaints procedure was drawn up in an attitude of defensiveness and was used as a device for filtering out and discouraging potential claims (Ackroyd 1986). The claimants' group Action for Victims of Medical Accidents suggested that the procedure was better designed to do this than to provide explanations to complainants as to what might have gone wrong. They argued that there was an undue emphasis on the fear of litigation and in their experience most complainants wanted information, an apology or an assurance that the same thing would not happen again rather than to sue (Simanowitz 1999).

There was strong evidence that a substantial number of complainants did not know how to make a complaint. In one study it was reported that in four districts surveyed only 5 per cent of members of the public questioned knew how to make a formal complaint (Prescott-Clarke et al. 1989). In line with such criticisms, the ACHCEW argued that, in its experience, few health authorities were fully meeting their obligations under current guidelines to publicize their complaints procedures (ACHCEW 1990).[15] The Audit Commission found that 45 per cent of the wards visited by its representatives did not have any posted or written information about the complaints system (Audit Commission 1993). Part of the problem was that guidelines operating at the time required, among other things, that information about how to complain should not be displayed in hospital wards lest it encourage patients to make 'unfounded' or 'frivolous' complaints.[16] It was also suggested that, despite some evidence of good practice, NHS procedures were often ineffective in meeting complainants' objectives. Several commentators highlighted the lack of satisfaction with the procedure among complainants (Donaldson and Cavanagh 1992; Lloyd-Bostock and Mulcahy 1994; Scottish Management Executive 1994).

There was also research evidence that suggested that complainants' needs were not being served. It was argued that replies to complainants continued to appear defensive despite the hope of the Davies Committee that this approach was to be discouraged. In their review of 71 letters of response to appeal-stage complainants, Donaldson and Cavanagh (1992: 24) commented:

Our experience is that complaints are not welcomed by health service managers or doctors. At best they tend to be greeted neutrally, but we have found that they are regarded by some doctors as an affront to their professional standing, and on occasions there has been talk of action being initiated by the doctor concerned on the grounds of defamation.

Similarly, in the words of Kaye and MacManus (1990: 1254):

> We can easily sympathise with . . . defensive responses, but all too
> frequently this initial reflex dominates the subsequent handling
> of the complaint and fails to either treat the complainant as an
> individual customer or identify and respond to the substance of
> the complaint. This sequence regularly produces an exchange of
> written denials or evasions resulting in mutual frustration. Thus the
> form is observed – the complaint is 'dealt with' – but the essence is
> denied.

Critics were also concerned about the lack of information on how
independent reviews worked. Most evidence suggested that the independent
review could be a daunting experience for the complainant. A number were
deterred from using the procedure because it could involve meeting the very
clinician being complained about. Complainants also voiced fears of being
victimized or labelled as troublesome by clinical staff (Lloyd-Bostock and
Mulcahy 1994). Moreover, the operation of the procedure lacked consistency. Complainants had no *right* to a review. Rather, the Regional Director
of Public Health had a discretion to decide whether an IPR was appropriate
and it was suggested that some directors were unwilling to exercise their
discretion in favour of the complainant (ACHCEW 1990). Statistics on the
use of the IPR certainly illustrate great diversity of practice between regions.
Regions such as Anglia and Oxford had conducted less than a fifth of the
number of reviews carried out in other regions over the period 1985–91.
The result was not only that a review would not always be granted, but that
a complainant might succeed in securing a review in one region where a
similar case might not be sent for review in another. Delays in resolving
complaints were also apparent. The IPR came at a very late stage in the complaints process and a complaint could take as long as three years to get
there. By the time the case was heard, the complainant would have had
to go over the history of the case at least three or four times in a formal
setting.[17]

The decision to call the review 'independent' was also considered a
peculiar one. It was suggested that:

> features of the peer review process call into question whether the
> process is intended to be an objective investigation of the complaint
> and whether it will be perceived as such by the complainant. More-
> over, they perhaps further highlight the ambiguity about whether
> the procedure is perceived as addressing the patient problem or
> addressing the needs of a problem patient.
>
> (Donaldson and Cavanagh 1992: 24–5)

The ability of the assessors to deliver an independent assessment was also called into question. Donaldson and Cavanagh (1992) found that the proportion of complaints upheld at IPR stage varied significantly by category of allegation. Most of the variation was due to a higher proportion of complaints about communication being upheld than those involving the application of clinical skill. They suggested that communication and behaviour complaints were seen as less threatening aspects of professional practice on which peers could rebuke a colleague. Finally, the procedure was shrouded in mystery and largely invisible. Discussions between the consultants after the review were confidential. They were required to send a copy of their report to the regional medical officer who would then instruct district personnel to reply to the complainant. But the complainant had no right to see the report and no chance to question the judgement of the reviewers. In some cases, complainants were merely being told that their case was not proven. Moreover, there were no immediate sanctions which could be taken against staff found responsible for an adverse event or occurrence, although recommendations can be made to the authority.

The new quality agenda

These various criticisms led to pressures on policy makers to revise the system in order to make it more 'consumer friendly'. The issue of how the necessity for change came to be identified is partially explained by a shift in the two main political parties' policy agenda towards quality. It could be argued that the newly found rhetoric of consumerism was used to legitimate policy initiatives which stressed the importance of quality mechanisms in the public sector. Significantly, complaints were seen as an important facet of quality data which could be used to facilitate public sector managers' quality and efficiency goals (Allsop and Mulcahy 1999). When the 1991 *Citizen's Charter* introduced a programme for the reform of public services, it had a significant impact on thinking about how complaints procedures should be designed. Each government department was required to produce a charter which listed entitlements, set performance targets and outlined mechanisms for the redress of grievances. But in addition, the original charter promised a further examination of complaints procedures and a review of public sector complaint systems was subsequently undertaken by the Cabinet Office Complaints Task Force. Three main themes run throughout the charter programme documentation on complaints. First, there was a concern to improve management within public services to make them more responsive to patient's needs. Second, there was a view that in monopoly services, where the opportunity for exit and using alternative services was limited, consumers should be encouraged to voice their concerns. Third, there was a belief that private sector business offered an appropriate model for learning from complaints (see e.g. Cabinet Office 1988; Cabinet Office Complaints Task Force 1993a, 1995a, 1995b).

In response to the criticisms of the existing procedure and the change in the policy making climate, the DoH set up its own inquiry into NHS complaints procedures in primary and secondary care under the chairmanship of Professor Alan Wilson (NHSE 1994).[18] The Wilson Committee, which reported in 1994, acknowledged that the procedure tended to favour the needs of staff over those of complainants. In particular, the Committee drew attention to the lack of knowledge about how to complain, the ways in which people were deterred from complaining, the lack of satisfactory responses and the ways in which the handling of complaints often appeared to increase the complainant's sense of grievance.[19] It was contended that 'Complainants can face an uphill struggle when using NHS complaints procedures: firstly in making their views known; and secondly, in receiving the sort of response they would wish for' (NHSE 1994: 20).

The Wilson Report's analysis of the problems encountered by users of the existing system lacks the depth of Sir Michael Davies' earlier report.[20] However, the Wilson Report and analysis of evidence presented to it does suggest that a range of different models of complaints handling were considered by the Committee including those based on tribunals, self-regulatory models (of the kind operated by the GMC), consumerist models, managerial-bureaucratic models (which placed emphasis on organizational needs) and various combinations of all the above. Despite this, their final choice of a managerial model can be seen as reformist rather than radical. An analysis of submissions to the committee by Moss and Stacey (1994) demonstrated that the committee veered towards this model despite the bulk of submissions favouring something more consumerist.[21]

The most important recommendations of the Wilson Committee for the purposes of the present work were that clinical and non-clinical complaints in both the primary and secondary care sectors should be dealt with under the same procedure. The reasoning for this reversal of previous policy seems to have been based on pragmatic rather than principled grounds as the quotation below suggests. It was contended that:

> We also think there is no need for a separate system for complaints about clinical judgement, whether of doctors or of other clinical staff . . . it is unhelpful to draw what is sometimes an artificial distinction between causes of particular concern, sometimes within a particular complaint. Complaints may, for example, be about facilities, behaviour or clinical practice, and often combinations of some, or all of these. It can be confusing if these are handled under separate procedures.
>
> (NHSE 1994: 40)

In this way, the Committee's recommendations paved the way for the abolition of the self-regulated appeals procedure which operated in hospitals. In its place the Committee recommended a panel made up of lay people *advised* by clinicians.

Current systems

Following on from the publication of the Wilson Committee report, a new NHS complaints procedure was introduced from April 1996. The guidance issued from the NHS Executive reflected the fashion for a 'rolling back' of the state and increasing the discretion of local providers. In line with this approach the procedure was not prescriptive about how health organizations should conduct the process of local resolution. Instead, emphasis was placed on the principles which should guide good practice, such as openness, flexibility, fairness and understanding what complainants want. What is most significant about this system today is that it continues to place considerable emphasis on the handling of complaints by practitioners at local level. Despite the increased formality of 'appeals' procedures, consultants are now actively encouraged to manage their own complaints.

The Wilson Committee was responsible for the introduction of the two key principles which were to guide the drafting of the new guidelines. First, that grievances are best resolved at local level by those responsible for the provision of the service being complained about. Second, that appeals from local resolution should only be made available in exceptional circumstances and that the discretion to set up an appeal should rest with a locally-based NHS employee. It is clear from the guidelines that emerged that the Committee and NHS Executive placed considerable faith in the ability of local providers to deal with complaints effectively. While recognizing the need for both formal and informal elements in complaint handling, a major tenet of the new procedures is that in the majority of cases resolution and satisfaction can be achieved most effectively by the provision of rapid, personal and informal responses to complaints. The new guidelines require Trusts, GP practices and health authorities to develop a simplified two-stage structure for complaint handling. At stage one, complaint handling is seen as the responsibility of those being complained about with a view to early resolution. Practice-based procedures are described as being practice-owned and managed. Complaints are seen as the responsibility of all staff and training in complaints handling has been recommended for all NHS staff likely to be in contact with patients. There is a certain common sense logic to this approach. Misunderstandings can most easily be identified and responded to at this level. Moreover, when provided at service level, remedies have the potential to seem more genuine since they are not forced following adjudication on the issue.

Stage one displays many of the hallmarks of informality. The guidelines are not prescriptive about the precise nature of procedures to be adopted, although they must comply with minimum national standards relating to publicity of the procedure and the provision of a structured and timely reply. The guidelines place emphasis on principles rather than procedures: flexibility and understanding what the complainant wants are key issues. They suggest that rigid, bureaucratic and legalistic approaches should be avoided at all stages of the procedure, but particularly during local resolution. The procedures also allow for the use of conciliators in the resolution of complaints, although, like the terms of service which governed primary care complaints before April 1996, the new guidance is rather vague about how such conciliation should be conducted and how suitable conciliators are to be trained or appointed. This approach is in marked contrast to the use of conciliation or mediation in many other fields where there is intense debate about the advantages of different mediatory models and the level of qualifications required of mediators. It is also somewhat surprising, given the launch of the DoH's medical negligence mediation pilot scheme a year prior to the introduction of the new complaints procedures, that greater thought was not given to how the two schemes connected and what lessons could be learned from the national mediation agencies about the value of training and accreditation.

At stage two of the procedure, dissatisfied complainants can refer their grievance to a convener who has the discretion to decide whether an IPR should be set up. Where insufficient attempts have been made at local resolution the convener can refer the case back to the first stage. Where the decision is made not to convene a panel, the convener is under a duty to give clear reasons for their decision. Where a panel is called, it is chaired by an independent chair nominated from a regional list, and staffed by the convener and (where the complaint involves a Trust), a representative of the purchaser. If the complaint involves clinical care, then two independent clinical assessors must be appointed.

At about the same time as the Wilson reforms were being introduced, changes were also brought about in the jurisdiction of the HSC. In the past, the HSC was only able to receive complaints about failures of service and maladministration as far as they related to non-clinical matters in the hospital sector. From April 1996, the HSC's role was extended to include grievances concerned with clinical judgement, services provided by general medical, ophthalmic or pharmaceutical practitioners or matters relating to family health service authority service committee hearings. The HSC has predicted, on the basis of his experience since the expansion of his jurisdiction, that in future the majority of complaints which his office investigates will involve clinical matters and will require clinical advice (HSC 1997–8).

The new procedures reflect a significant shift in the policy emphasis. First, an important jurisdictional shift has occurred in the control of the second tier of the procedure and review by the HSC. The new procedure places responsibility for setting up and reporting of panel decisions squarely within the jurisdiction of managers and bureaucrats. Chairs of panels are selected from the laity and they receive advice from clinical assessors but do not have to be bound by it. As far as the HSC is concerned there has been an acceptance at policy level of the argument that the HSC is capable of making decisions about the appropriateness of clinical judgements as long as they are able to employ their own clinical advisers. Second, key decisions makers, most notably the chair and convener, are accountable to complainants and managers for their decisions and have a duty to give reasons for them. Finally, an attempt has been made to simplify the various channels for complaints by uniting the primary and secondary sector within a common framework for complaint handling.

How well is the new procedure working? Three research studies have investigated the post-1996 complaint system (see Kyffin et al. 1997; Wallace and Mulcahy 1999), one of which was an official evaluation commissioned by the DoH (2001). Evidence from all three studies indicates a number of sources of dissatisfaction with both the local resolution stage and the Independent Review Panel (IRP) process. Despite the different methodologies adopted, the findings of the studies are broadly in agreement about the reasons for dissatisfaction. The first independent evaluation of the new procedure undertaken by the Public Law Project (PLP) (Wallace and Mulcahy 1999) shows that while local resolution can work well, complainants and their representatives are concerned about the lack of impartiality and visibility.[22] While managers have generally expressed satisfaction with the new procedures for local resolution, data from the national surveys Wallace and Mulcahy conducted suggested that there were inherent weaknesses in the local resolution process. Its informality and flexibility was thought to allow too much scope for grievances to be handled in inappropriate ways when viewed from a complaints perspective.[23] There was also a perceived failure to take sufficient account of the imbalance of power in the health professional-patient relationship. In particular, it was felt that those involved in local resolution often failed to recognize how difficult it can be to complain. Participants in the research also reported that, while local resolution expected the parties to a dispute to be open, honest and trusting, in truth service-level disputes were often emotionally charged and the parties suspicious of each other.

The PLP research has also shown that there are weaknesses in how local resolution is being conducted. Around two-thirds of respondents were dissatisfied with: the fairness of the process which was seen as biased in favour of staff; the poor attitude of complaint handlers; and the inadequacies of results. Conveners in the PLP survey sent back nearly half (47 per cent) of the cases referred to them for further local resolution. In many cases this was because inappropriate responses had been made to complainants by those involved in the complaint or because inadequate investigations had been conducted.

The same research revealed that the ways in which IRPs are established and conducted did not give complainants confidence in their independence or effectiveness in holding the NHS to account. There was a lack of transparency in the ways in which the panels were conducted which suggest that the principles of due process are still not being fully satisfied. For example, the parties to the complaint typically were seen separately by adjudicators and given no opportunity to question each other about their accounts and explanations. Panel hearings were rarely held on neutral premises and were sometimes administered by the same staff who were involved in local resolution.

The same research has suggested that complainants are doubtful about whether their complaint would help to raise the quality of services, although one of the main reasons for complaining may be to prevent the same thing happening to someone else. While many health organizations endeavour to use complaints for quality management, this is often hampered by fragmentary coordination of data from these and other sources of information – for example, audit and adverse clinical incidents. Despite the recommendations of the Wilson Committee that complaints should be recorded and used for quality and risk management, little guidance has been given and a national classification system for complaints has not been developed. The data that providers are required to send to the DoH do not break down the largest single category, clinical complaints, into further subsets and GPs are not required to give information on complaints made to them. Furthermore, in their study of 12 Trusts, Kyffin et al. (1997) argue that oral complaints are often not recorded at all and that complainants' letters which contain a number of allegations are, in practice, reduced to a single category.

The PLP research and the HSC's reports have also highlighted concerns about the convening role and the ability of conveners to establish an impartial stance (HSC 1996–7, 1997–8, 1998–9, 1999–2000, 2000–1). Almost half (46 per cent) of the 169 conveners in the PLP survey felt that their independence was compromised by existing links to the health care provider and a number were also concerned that they did not have a sufficient caseload to have gained enough experience of the role. The research drew particular attention to conveners' and IRP chairs' concerns that they were stepping beyond their formal remit and trying to resolve complaints. Such activity can appear confusing to complainants who may have been led to expect a greater element of impartiality at this stage of the procedure.

Perhaps most significantly, commentators have expressed concerns that the new procedures have encouraged the privatization of justice by legitimating service-level handling of complaints without adequate checks on whether complaints are being handled well (Mulcahy and Allsop 1997). Although attempts at visibility have been made by policy makers, these have concentrated on the second stage of the procedure designed to deal with the small minority of complaints which can be taken further in the procedure at the discretion of conveners. For doctors, the new arrangements for complaints handling appear to have considerable benefits. Staff, including doctors and their professional associations were included in the complaints system evaluation study *Handling Complaints* (DoH 2001). In contrast to complainants, a much larger proportion of NHS staff were satisfied with the new procedures. Around two-thirds thought that the complaint was handled well and that it was dealt with within the time limits. Staff found that their colleagues had been supportive through the process and that the process was fair and unbiased although more than half of the respondents were not satisfied with the way they were kept informed of the progress of the complaint and almost three-quarters said they found the process stressful.

New emphasis has been placed on the privacy of dispute resolution, especially where local resolution and conciliation are used. But concern has been expressed that the new procedures do little to enhance the power of patients and their relatives who are still in the weaker position of being at the receiving end of a largely monopolistic service. The procedures reveal an ongoing tension between the needs of complainants, doctors, managers and the general public. In the words of Mulcahy (1999: 81):

> While the new guidance employs the rhetoric of consumerism and managerialism, it may actually have reinforced self-regulation by encouraging complaint handling to go underground at practice level. Complaints may be being handled in an exemplary fashion . . . but how do we know whether this is the case?

Conclusion

This chapter has suggested that the fortunes of the hospital complaints procedure have closely mirrored ongoing debate about doctors' claims to clinical autonomy. Concessions to the idea of the closer involvement of the state in the regulation of the profession have been made and have served to reiterate the point that the authority of the medical profession in terms of self-regulation and clinical autonomy derives from the state. The profession has conceded that there should be a hospital complaints procedure, formulated by the executive body of the NHS, which operates in parallel to the GMC's own procedure. They have agreed that the hospital procedure should have an 'appeals' process which is removed from service level. But in many other ways the claim to clinical autonomy and self-regulation has been successful. The profession managed to limit for many years the operation of the 'appeals' procedure to include only medics in the review process and to fashion it as a medical consultation rather than a legal procedure. Moreover, the discretion to instigate change as a result of a finding of fault was left in the hands of the senior medical officer at regional level. The procedure which operated until 1996 was very different from the tribunal-like structure recommended by Sir Michael Davies. Moreover, throughout the development of the procedure there has been minimal monitoring of complaints at service level and somewhat ambiguous provisions about the reporting of complaints. In terms of accessibility the shift to a more managerial model for dealing with complaint systems has brought greater openness. It is also possible that the encouragement of a variety of approaches to resolution has encouraged more participatory forms. However, it is likely that the large element of discretion in how to proceed has brought considerable variation.

The new procedures reveal a tension between the needs of individual complainants, providers of medical services and the needs of the general public and the state in regulating medical work. In complaints, particularly those which are not readily resolved, there may be differing accounts, different perceptions and different interests at stake. Underlying these difficulties there are issues of power. The regulation of professional groups in society is a complex task. Indeed, the health service reforms deliberately delegate authority for decision making and regulation downwards. While procedures have brought all groups within the managerial remit in the Trust sector, the large element of discretion and the lack of requirements to meet particular standards or provide information about complaints put the onus back on complainants to pursue their concerns.

There is also the issue of accountability. The intention of modern procedures was that health authorities and Trusts should investigate, record and analyse complaints and use the information to improve practice. As May (1998: 21) suggests: 'Despite all the rhetoric about involving the public, there is strangely little recognition that complaints handling is the crossroads where public involvement, clinical audit and managerial performance come together'. There are minimal requirements for reporting back either to the boards of Trusts or to health authorities, let alone to communities or the general public. Even with the shift away from the rigours of a contracting culture, the political sensitivity of health care encourages secretiveness at a local and national level which inhibits an open approach to complaint handling.

The 1997 White Paper on the NHS, *The New NHS* (DoH 1997), and the consultative document *A First Class Service* (DoH 1998) put an emphasis on a variety of new measures to develop further a culture in the NHS committed to achieving high clinical standards as well as efficiency through 'clinical governance' – a comprehensive system of monitoring and review which will operate at all levels of the service. However, the Secretary of State commented in the White Paper: 'The Government will continue to work with the professions, the regulatory bodies, the NHS and patient representative groups to strengthen the existing systems of professional self-regulation by ensuring that they are open, responsive and publicly accountable' (DoH 1997: 59). In the future, as well as in the past, self-regulation is seen as the key to achieving these goals. Considerable vigilance will be required by all the stakeholders in health care to ensure that a balance is struck between protecting the health service user and supporting the clinical professions in the process of managing their grievances.

Notes

1   There are procedures in place to allow for the suspension of doctors working for NHS hospitals based on the contract of employment. However, these are extremely convoluted and are rarely used. Of course, this means that their contract can be terminated if they are in breach of its provisions but this mechanism is an unwieldy regulatory tool and is not well suited to dealing with minor and moderate transgressions.
2   Although doctors' contracts were negotiated centrally by politicians, bureaucrats and medico-politicos such as the GMC and BMA.
3   NHS Reorganisation Act 1973.
4   The terms of reference of the Davies Committee were: 'To provide the hospital service with practical guidance in the form of a code of principles and practice for recording and investigating matters affecting patients which go wrong in hospitals; for receiving complaints or suggestions by patients, staff or others about such matters; and for communicating the results of investigations; and to make recommendations' (DHSS 1973).
5   The final report of the Committee is 163 pages long.
6   The 16 places on the Davies Committee were occupied by senior administrators (4), academics (3), senior medics (3), representatives of consumer organizations (2), journalists (2), an NHS trade unionist and a senior nurse.
7   It commissioned research by the Institute for Operational Research. This involved a survey of 455 former in-patients and 558 former out-patients and case studies at five individual hospitals.
8   Responses were received from all the regional hospital boards, 64 per cent of boards of governors (21), 91 per cent of hospital management committees and boards of governors (302) and 49 per cent of other organizations and individuals approached for evidence. As a result of a widespread publicity campaign, an additional 859 letters were received from members of the public.
9   Several years later the Minister of State for Health and Social Security was to assert that at the time the only real alternative to internal resolution of complaints was to go to the courts (DHSS 1983b). More complaints appeared to filter through to members of the hospital authority than to regional boards, especially where they involved clinicians, but evidence submitted to the committee suggested that in the majority of cases members of health authorities decided that no further action was necessary.

10 Unfortunately, the Davies Report does not distinguish between professional and head of department when presenting the data.

11 The Committee recommended the setting-up of a separate grievance procedure to deal with disputes of this kind. If cases could not be resolved in this way, it was suggested that they should be referred to the chair of the medical advisory committee and then on to external medical advisers. Thus, while it recognized the tension between the responsibilities of bureaucrats and medics, it conceded that the final arbiter of such disputes should be a medic.

12 The Bill received all-party backing but three objections to it were reported in parliamentary debate. The first two of these reflect a concern about the impact of complaints. The BMA argued that existing procedures were adequate to deal with complaints. The second objection came from the Confederation of Health Service Employees which supported the Bill but wanted reassurance that any new procedures would give their members adequate time to prepare a defence to any allegation. The third objection came from Baroness Marsham of Ion who argued that the Bill should include a provision that complainants would not suffer any disadvantage as a result of making a complaint. Her suggested amendment was withdrawn when Lord Caithness argued that this was an impossible area on which to legislate and an undertaking was given that a suitable provision would be included instead in guidance to health authorities on the operation of the Act.

13 Attention has also been drawn to the fact that allegations of bad practice in the handling of complaints by health authorities comprised about one-sixth of the workload of the HSC in 1989–90 (Donaldson and Cavanagh 1992).

14 This view has been repeated by many. See, for example, Action for Victims of Medical Accidents, *Lawyers Service Newsletter*, March 1988.

15 Instead of producing special leaflets providing information on how to complain, many relied on sections inserted into patient information booklets. The ACHCEW argued that not only did this make the information less accessible, it meant that those using out-patient, accident and emergency and long-term residential care did not receive the information at all.

16 Dame Elizabeth Ackroyd, Chair of the Patients Association, argued that, no doubt, some complaints did deserve such epithets but that such prejudgement should not be made about all complainants (Ackroyd 1986).

17 In a review of 171 cases considered for IPRs, Geffen (1990) found that the time taken to handle them was from six months to over two years.

18 The Committee, which was made up of a mix of businesspeople, academics and consumer groups had the unenviable task of steering a course between the needs of complainants, staff, managers and policy makers.

19 Their views were not universally supported as was made clear by their recognition that the JCC, despite considerable evidence to the contrary, continued to maintain that the clinical complaints procedure satisfied the needs of complainants.

20   Unlike the Davies Committee which had reported 20 years earlier, the Wilson Committee did not take extensive evidence, conduct research or deliberate at length. Committee meetings were all held over seven months. In contrast to the Davies Report, Wilson made proposals for the broad features of the new complaints procedures but suggested that the implementation and operation should be left to individual organizations in order to allow them to tailor processes to suit local conditions.

21   The Committee also took the unprecedented step of developing a checklist of general principles which ought to govern reform of the procedure. These were: responsiveness; quality enhancement; cost-effectiveness; accessibility; impartiality; simplicity; speed; confidentiality; and accountability. The majority of these standards reflect the requirements of natural justice but the managerialist political culture of the time is also reflected in the emphasis on quality enhancement.

22   Some were sceptical about whether they would receive an open and fair explanation from those directly involved in their care and many feared that they might suffer some form of retribution. The HSC has deplored the fact that some GPs have asked patients, and sometimes their families as well, to leave their practice following a complaint. It has been recommended that changes be made to the GP contract so that GPs must give reasons for removing a patient.

23   In *Handling Complaints* (DoH 2001), complaint managers said they thought the new process was more impartial, more flexible and encouraged learning from complaints compared to the system prior to 1996. However, they also thought that changes were needed to make the system easier to operate. The chief executives in the study believed that local resolution was more cost effective. A large majority (85 per cent) said that they had met face-to-face with complainants – a finding that contradicts that of complainants who felt there were too few meetings. Chief executives were most critical of the performance targets set and particularly of the time limits, which were seen as most unrealistic.

4   The phantom menace?

Looking at the relationship between
medical mishaps, complaints and
negligence claims

Introduction

This chapter seeks to place this study of complaints in the context of other
phenomena with which complaints have a connection. It considers how medical mishaps, dissatisfaction with health care, complaints and medical negligence claims are conceptualized and how the links between them are best
understood. Although interest in these activities has increased in recent years,
few scholars have attempted to understand the relationship between them
(but see Annandale and Hunt 1998; Mulcahy and Tritter 1998). As with
previous chapters the concern here is with considering how these terms have
come to be understood. The analysis presented places particular emphasis on
the influences wielded by the medical profession in defining these terms. It
is argued that terms such as 'error', 'dissatisfaction' and 'grievance' are not
natural events which occur outside of the language which describes them.
Instead, they are the products of language which reflect power relations in the
doctor-patient relationship and dominant ways of thinking. The discussion in
this chapter draws on a number of largely discrete literatures which deal with
the notions of error, dissatisfaction with health care, complaining and legal
claims. The commentaries on these subjects which have taken place have
occurred in the different spheres of law, medical sociology, social psychology
and anthropology. In drawing on this diverse range of materials the chapter
raises a number of issues around whose values should inform the definition of
medical harm, what constitutes 'appropriate' care or an 'acceptable' risk and
what constitutes sufficient cause to complain or claim.

It is noticeable that those interested in the evolution of grievances have
tended to see expressions of dissatisfaction as potential complaints which in
turn are potential claims rather than discrete phenomena (see e.g. Fitzgerald
and Dickens 1980–1). Despite this, the importance of understanding dissatisfaction which is not pursued to the end of this pathway has not been ignored.
Felstiner et al. argue that a 'theory that looked only at institutions mobilized

by disputants and the strategies pursued within them would be seriously deficient. It would look like constructing a theory of politics entirely on the basis of the voting patterns when we know that most people do not vote in most elections' (1980–1: 636). While the occurrence of a medical mishap may lead to dissatisfaction and a voiced grievance, it is clear from research that the vast majority do not. My own understanding of the relationship between these discrete but related concepts is shown in Figure 4.1. This chapter attempts to unravel ways in which the phenomena represented in the figure relate, and the various ways in which they are distinct from each other.

A key theme to emerge from this chapter is the many ways in which our inclination is to look for someone to blame when something goes wrong. This is somewhat curious as recent research suggests that the majority of medical mishaps are caused by systemic failures – a chain of associated actions by a variety of people. Emphasis on the individualization of responsibility is compounded by complaints and litigation systems which are hostile to complaints raised by groups of people. What do these characteristics tell us about the ways in which the aftermath of medical mishap is managed? Whose interests are best served by such management of risk? The chapter begins with an analysis of each of the key concepts referred to above and considers the relationships, or perceived relationships, between mishaps, dissatisfaction and grievances.

Key concepts

The notion of medical mishap

Various terms have been chosen to designate inappropriate care and adverse outcomes experienced by patients. These include adverse or untoward events, maloccurrences, complications, medical injuries, therapeutic misadventures, substandard care, unexpected outcomes, preventable deaths, iatrogenic injury, mishaps, errors, negligence or malpractice.[1] These various definitions

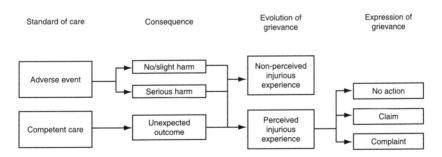

Figure 4.1   Journeys to complaints and medical negligence claims (after Felstiner et al. 1980–1)

often reveal something of the context in which they are used. But they also reveal assumptions about claims to knowledge and expertise. Andrews et al. (1997) have argued that one of the main reasons why studies of adverse events underestimate the incidence of medical mishap is because it requires two physicians to agree that an adverse event occurred.[2]

The terminology of medical mishap is culturally specific and has changed over time. But it was not until the incidence of claims began to rise in the 1960s in the West that interest was aroused in the incidence of error, and serious attention was not given to the matter until the aftermath of the medical litigation 'crisis' in the USA in the 1970s. In subsequent treatments of the subject different lay and medical definitions have emerged and these reflect different epistemologies of health and illness. Doctors' definitions of medical error have been particularly influential and once again this can be explained by recourse to the principles which underline the notion of state-sanctioned and self-regulation. If it is only doctors who have the skills and knowledge to undertake medical procedures then it might be argued that it is only doctors who can determine when a mishap has occurred. This gives doctors a definitional power denied to the laity. In turn this affords doctors political power in public debate about error, allowing the profession to argue for instance that, with the growth of new technologies, iatrogenic injury in modern times has been understood as the inevitable price of medical progress, part of the sequelae of sound and sanctioned medical practice (Sharpe and Faden 1998; Smith 1999). Doctors also have situational power as they are best able to control the visibility of error and its effects, and help determine a patient's initial response.

These broader conceptualizations clearly have a role to play in the everyday handling of mishap. Bosk's (1979) important study of the management of error in two surgical units suggests that the way in which mishap is constructed will radically effect the amount and type of error which professionals perceive. Research undertaken in the USA has shown that untoward events in diagnosis and treatment tend to be redefined not as mistakes or errors but as part of the inherent risk of undertaking medical treatment (Bosk 1979; Mizrahi 1984). This conceptualization has been supported by those who tend to see medicine as an art rather than an exact science. The presentation of risk and mishap may also rely on prevalent views about the level of information doctors think it appropriate to reveal to patients. Christakis (1999) argued that prognosis poses particular difficulties because of the perceived need among medical staff in his qualitative study to give positive messages to patients and relatives. Participants in the study argued that what some see as under-reporting reflects a misunderstanding of the medical encounter. The doctors in this study reinforced the view that the moral norms governing such activity should come from inside the canons of professional practice or science.

While the terminology of medical mishaps seems to be contested there appears to be agreement that even if narrowly defined by doctors the incidence is significant. In recent years a number of studies, most of which have focused on the hospital sector in the USA, have revealed that the occurrence of medical mishaps is sizeable and much higher than would be tolerated in hazardous industries such as aviation and nuclear power.[3] The most famous and comprehensive study undertaken to date is the Harvard Medical Malpractice Study (Leape et al. 1991) which reported the results of a review of 30,121 medical records in New York State.[4] This revealed that nearly 4 per cent of patients suffered an injury which prolonged their hospital stay or resulted in a measurable disability. Nearly 14 per cent of these injuries were fatal. If these rates are typical of the USA then approximately 18,000 people are likely to die there each year as a result of iatrogenic injury, making preventable adverse events the eighth leading cause of death there. Still higher figures have been obtained in older research projects,[5] studies of elderly patients[6] and in a recent Australian study in which 17 per cent of admissions led to a medical mishap (Wilson et al. 1995; Thomas and Brennan 2000; see also Andrews et al. 1997). In a UK setting Vincent (1995) found in a smaller-scale pilot study that 7 per cent of hospital patients were the subject of medical mishaps. He concluded that this led to a mean of seven extra days in hospital for those involved, at a cost of £67,000 for 500 cases.[7]

One of the problems with the identification and tracking of medical mishaps and near misses is that they are not always reported. Does this occur as a result of disagreement about what constitutes a medical mishap or as a result of attempts to conceal error? The Harvard study indicated that many medical mishaps noted on the medical record and deemed by medical researchers as negligent were not acted upon (Brennan et al. 1991). Andrews et al.'s (1997) prospective observational study of the work rounds and clinical meetings of 1047 surgery patients in a selection of US hospitals found that at least one unreported error was identified in the care of 44 per cent of the patients. In some of these cases it is likely that an error was simply not spotted. In others it may well be the case that problems have been identified but reporting rejected as a possible course of action. Drawing on his own empirical studies, Christakis (1999) has argued that doctors tend to be underprepared for truth-telling in their training and fear a loss of status with colleagues and patients if they are seen to be getting things wrong. The Bristol Inquiry (2001) identified a number of other barriers to reporting medical mishaps including a culture of blame and punishment; the assumption of perfectibility; a code of silence; and fear of clinical negligence systems based on establishing blame and fault.

The notion of dissatisfaction

What about the impact on patients? How often are patients aware of mishaps in their treatment and how do they respond? In contrast to the discussion of mishap above the stories of error told by dissatisfied patients, complainants and claimants do not reflect a belief that harm is an inevitable consequence of medical practice, nor do they accept that it is only doctors who have the skill and knowledge to identify mishap. They stress instead the violations of professional standards and lack of attention to the dignity and autonomy of the patient, their relatives and friends. Emphasis is also placed on the experiential knowledge of patients.

Sociologists have done much to enhance our understanding of how dissatisfaction is constructed within particular social settings and how professional dominance can inhibit the questioning of doctors' judgement (Stimson and Webb 1975; Strong and Davis 1977; Annandale and Hunt 1998). Recent investigations have shown that the presumption of trust is strongly embedded in people's perceptions of clinical acts. As a result, it can take a considerable time for a person to interpret the behaviour of a health professional as potentially injurious. This has been vividly portrayed in the Bristol Inquiry (2001) and in the CHI (2001) report on the Loughborough GP, Peter Green. One of the most haunting aspects of the Shipman Inquiry has been the revelation that so many of his patients had continued to place trust in him despite his homicidal activities. In addition to trust, structural factors such as social class, patriarchy, ethnicity and deviance have been identified as creating environments in which dissatisfaction remains unperceived (Goffman 1971; Nader 1980; Oakley 1980; Cornwall 1984; Littlewood and Lipsedge 1989; Foucault 1973).

In his telephone interviews with 547 US health consumers, Andreasen (1985) argued that perceiving dissatisfaction in loose monopolies is a function of three factors: the opportunity to experience dissatisfaction; the ability to detect it; and the motivation to look for it. Ability to detect dissatisfaction is clearly affected by the extent to which doctors and patients have a shared understanding of the condition experienced, appropriate treatment of it and what should occur in the aftermath of medical intervention. In a society such as ours, where medical 'science' is highly specialized, patients will experience particular problems when they lack information or understanding about scientific data or models to detect inappropriate treatment (Hopkins 1993). Hunt (1991) has argued that we live in a world where we are increasingly incompetent to judge what is appropriate in a medical context because of the rise of medical technology. This modern development serves to widen the divide between experts and laity and also reinforces a scientific model of medicine.

The problems involved in recognizing mishap may be self-induced by patients not asking the right questions or may be externally manipulated – for example, when information about inadequate services is deliberately withheld by an organization or carer. Even when dissatisfaction emerges it remains a complex concept. Dissatisfaction may evolve from recognition of a medical mishap but it may just as easily come about as a result of a misplaced *perception* that something has gone wrong with the care received.[8] Making the same point in the context of complaining, one complaints manager has suggested:

> Some people complain only reluctantly and as a last resort, when prompted by a deep emotion. Some people complain reasonably on reasonable grounds. Some complain 'unreasonably' on reasonable grounds. Some complain 'reasonably' on unreasonable grounds. A few seem to be 'born complainants' who relish a battle and will complain on any grounds whatsoever.
>
> (Truelove 1985: 24)

It would seem then, that a causal link between dissatisfaction and a technical mishap is far from inevitable.

Patients and their relatives may also react to a perceived injurious experience in different ways. Carmel's (1988) study of Israeli hospital patients' responses to dissatisfaction found that power resources, perception of social power and situational power contribute to explanations of the intensity of response to concern about a possible error or inappropriate care. So, for example, those who made use of formal channels to express their dissatisfaction were likely to have stayed in hospital longer and perceive themselves as being in control.[9] Dissatisfaction may also manifest itself in unpredictable ways. Research has shown that many patients do not feel confident in assessing the skills of health professionals and may choose instead to focus their dissatisfaction on criticisms of non-medical aspects of care such as hotel services or bedside manner (Ben-Sira 1976; Fitzpatrick and Hopkins 1983). Finally, the very term 'dissatisfaction' has prompted debate. Studies of dissatisfaction have become common but as the literature develops it is becoming increasingly clear that the term cannot accommodate the range of feelings, beliefs and values people express when they encounter problems in health care. Coyle (1999) has suggested that notions of personal identity threat, disempowerment, dehumanization and devaluation are much more apt descriptions of the emotional context in which dissatisfaction must be placed.

The measurement of dissatisfaction with health services has become popular with policy makers and managers. But using patient surveys as a form of performance indicator, though laudable, is problematic. Once again, the methodologies employed will reflect particular conceptions of the doctor-patient relationship, as well as what constitutes appropriate care. Commentators' concerns have focused on the ways in which data about dissatisfaction has been collected. It has been argued that dominant definitions of consumer satisfaction and dissatisfaction, which compare what was expected with what was received, are overly simplistic. Hunt (1991) suggests a number of alternative ways of determining what might cause dissatisfaction including an assessment of whether what is received is culturally acceptable or the gain for the patient is more than is lost. Moreover, he argues that outcome, whether adverse or positive, should not be privileged as an indication of satisfaction. This is because the *process* of receiving treatment may be just as important a stimulus for the emergence of dissatisfaction. A technologically sophisticated patient may, for instance, appreciate that a doctor has carried out a treatment competently even if there is an adverse outcome.[10] In their critique of notions of dissatisfaction, Mulcahy and Tritter (1998) argued that people are much more willing to express satisfaction than dissatisfaction and that expressions of dissatisfaction tend to be much easier to categorize because they are much more focused.[11] Many other socio-legal scholars have emphasized the difficulty of researching and recording dissatisfaction, involving as it does 'ambiguous behaviour, faulty recall, uncertain norms, conflicting objectives, inconsistent values and complex institutions' (Felstiner et al. 1980–1). Expressions of dissatisfaction have been viewed as dynamic, fluid, responsive and difficult to record, classify or interpret (Williams et al. 1998). Research even suggests that patients may not use the same languages as researchers in voicing their concerns, nor be prepared to be identified as dissatisfied (Fitzpatrick and Hopkins 1983).[12]

The notion of voiced grievances and complaints

Dissatisfaction about medical care can be distinguished from complaining and claiming in a number of ways. First of all, dissatisfaction may be voiced within social networks or in response to questions in patient satisfaction surveys, but concerns about treatment may just as easily be left unsaid. By way of contrast, socio-legal researchers have argued that complaints and claims can only be defined as instances of *voiced grievances*. Second, it has been suggested that blaming must also occur before dissatisfaction or the 'naming' of a problem can transform into a complaint or claim. More specifically, while dissatisfaction involves the identification or naming of a problem, the process of blaming is said to involve the attribution of fault for the problem to a particular individual. Again, this transformation from dissatisfaction to the attribution of blame is far from inevitable. Patients and their supporters may come to understand poor outcomes as the result of bad luck or the inevitable consequence of medical intervention (Felstiner et al. 1980–1).

The 'naming, blaming and claiming' model has been influential in law and society scholarship and has been useful in attempting to make distinctions between the key concepts being discussed in this chapter. Despite this, modern-day critics have also expressed concerns about the centrality of concepts of blame and culpability to the notion of calling to account. It has been suggested that the process of voicing a grievance may not always be as linear as many people believe. Lloyd-Bostock's work in particular has challenged the validity of such pathway models, resting as they do on placing attributions of fault in a time sequence where people first name, then blame, then claim (Lloyd-Bostock and Mulcahy 1994). She argues that we should not necessarily expect people to arrive at perceptions, judgements and decisions in a particular order. Her vision of such transformations is messier. She suggests that attribution of cause, fault or blame may be formed, changed or refined over time and may sometimes occur after a decision has been made to make a complaint or claim. Social anthropologists have also been hesitant to attribute transformations to a particular moment in time but have stressed the ways in which, even when voiced, a grievance and responses to it can expand and narrow as arguments are rehearsed and tested among social networks and other audiences (Mather and Yngvesson 1980–1; Black and Baumgartner 1983).

According to Lloyd-Bostock's analysis of disputes, some attributions of fault are actually precipitated by the prospect or initiation of a claim and crystallized by the process of complaining. In support of her argument she refers to Harris et al.'s (1984) study of the behaviour of personal injury victims which demonstrated that significant numbers of people attributed fault to one person and made a legal claim against another. Some participants in the study even embarked on a legal claim without holding anyone at fault. Echoes of these patterns of behaviour can also be found in medical negligence litigation. Indeed, the litigation system in the UK has traditionally encouraged such behaviour by making senior consulting staff responsible in litigation for the actions and omissions of junior doctors and nurses on their team. It is also likely that patients who are in danger of being time-barred from litigation file suit in haste with a much less well developed sense of fault than that anticipated by the pathway model. Finally, it is clear that a number of complainants and litigants voice dissatisfaction and protest without a clear sense of who might be responsible for what has happened to them. In my own survey of what 128 medical negligence litigants wanted to achieve by bringing a legal action, 45 per cent wanted an investigation and 29 per cent wanted to be told what had happened.[13] These findings suggest that medical negligence actions are far from being mature disputes. Indeed, many practitioners have argued that it is not until expert witness reports are available that the parties can be sure that they are in dispute at all (Mulcahy et al. 1999).

These debates suggest that grievances and their expression are complex concepts. Empirical research has also made clear that there are a number of practical barriers to voicing. May and DeMarco's (1986) study of patient decisions in the transformation of disputes in a US setting found that the more severe treatment or diagnostic problems were most likely to be pursued as a formal grievance but that the most frequent response to mishap was either doing nothing or changing doctors. In their study of dissatisfaction in general practice, only 25 per cent of disgruntled patients contacted the doctors involved and only 11 per cent contacted a lawyer. Mulcahy and Tritter (1998) found the link to be even more tenuous in their study of the relationship between dissatisfaction and the voicing of a grievance. In their analysis of the 326 cases in their dataset of 1637 householders, where the respondents had expressed their grievances outside their immediate circle of friends and family they found only a handful of these cases were likely to feature in formal complaint statistics. Just 3 respondents reported that they had begun a legal claim and 17 had approached a CHC for advice. Even then, there was no indication that a formal complaint had ensued as a result. In one other case the respondent had received a letter of explanation from the provider which suggested that a formal complaint had been made.

Studies of the link between medical negligence claims and medical mishaps have also found that claiming is an atypical response to medical mishap. Danzon's (1985) seminal study of the relationship between adverse events and medical negligence claims found that only 1 in 25 negligent injuries resulted in compensation through the malpractice system. The Harvard Medical Malpractice Study found that there were seven times as many medical mishaps as claims for compensation and about 14 adverse events for every paid claim (Leape et al. 1991). Similarly, Andrews et al. (1997) found in their broader-based ethnographic study that, even though 18 per cent of patients had adverse events during their care, only 13 (1 per cent) of the 1047 in the study made claims[14] (see also Miller and Sarat 1980–1; May and DeMarco 1986). Studies of the relationship between complaints and claims have also suggested that the 'danger' of complaints progressing to claims has been overstated (Mulcahy and Lloyd-Bostock 1992; Jost et al. 1993).[15]

It is also clear from empirical studies that many people do not express their grievance in a formal setting because they do not know how to, fear retribution and defensive responses or because they do not believe that it would make a difference to their lives or the lives of others (Mulcahy and Tritter 1998). A Market and Opinion Research Institute (MORI) survey (1997) found this view was particularly likely to be expressed by young men and older women. It has also been argued that a key reason why people do not complain about doctors is that they feel doubly vulnerable. If they are long-term sick or likely to need future care, they may feel that the risk of upsetting the doctor and jeopardizing that future care is too great. In an analysis of Scottish data, Annadale and Hunt (1998) found that patients tended not to make formal complaints when they had a long-term relationship with a service provider to preserve, particularly where there was no alternative provider. This is especially common in inner-city conurbations and remote rural districts where it is difficult to recruit new staff to hospitals and GP practices. On the basis of evidence from complainants and CHCs, the PLP report (Wallace and Mulcahy 1999) and the DoH's official evaluation of the 1996 complaints procedure (DoH 2001) it was reported that people found it particularly difficult to make a complaint about their GP, or GP practice, because of fear that they might be removed from the practice list. An earlier national MORI survey undertaken in 1995 on attitudes to complaints about public services also found that more people feared recrimination in the health services than in any other public sector service except the police.

Knowledge of legal process and support networks are clearly important to understanding the dynamics of voicing. Those who have access to pertinent knowledge on how to complain or what to complain about are clearly advantaged over those who do not. Anthropologists of law have placed much emphasis on the presence or absence of supporters in the transformation of disputes (Mather and Yngvesson 1980–1; Black and Baumgartner 1983). Ladinsky and Susmilch (1983: 5) refer to such people as 'brokers' and describe them as 'critical communication linkages in the sustenance and suppression of consumer disputes'. Drawing on this framework, May (1991) distinguishes between 'broker-companions' such as family and friends and 'broker-knowledgeables' who have ways of finding out whether there were deficiencies in care. In their empirical study, May and Stengel (1987) found that those who sue their doctors are much more likely to have the support of family and friends in pursuing a medical negligence action and to have made contact with medical or legal 'knowledgeables' than those who choose not to.[16] Moreover, Hickson et al.'s (1992) study of factors that prompted families to file malpractice claims following perinatal injuries also found that knowledgeable acquaintances had a significant impact on the decision to file a claim. In their study of 127 families, 33 per cent had such a 'knowledgeable'.

Evidence suggests that lack of knowledge about how and where to complain may still be a problem for some groups. When people were asked about their general knowledge of how to complain, the 1995 MORI survey found that one in three respondents said they did not know how to do so. Lack of knowledge was a particular problem for those on low incomes and the less well educated, and focus group findings indicated that ethnic minority women also had particular difficulties. A follow-up study in 1997 (MORI 1997) found that views of complaining about public services had changed little in the NHS, although the existence of charters had made some difference.[17]

So far I have emphasized the ways in which formal systems can make themselves inaccessible to those with grievances about medical care. But there are many other reasons why dissatisfaction and grievances do not evolve into complaints or claims, which have nothing to do with the hostility of the legal system. Patients may also *choose* not to make a complaint or clinical negligence claim. In their study of the link between dissatisfaction and voiced grievances, Mulcahy and Tritter (1998) found that, for some, avoiding disputes is a positive and rational choice. Asked why they had not voiced their dissatis-faction, this subset said they had other priorities, wished to put negative experiences behind them or avoid confrontation. Stimson and Webb (1975) also found that conflict is generally contained and that patients find it more natural to cope with dissatisfaction through gossip networks and storytelling rather than discussing it with their doctor. These images are far removed from that of the overly litigious patient.

The notion of claiming

Socio-legal accounts of disputes define claiming as the voicing of a grievance to someone with responsibility to respond to it. Clearly, this definition is broad enough to encompass 'voicing' to any state-sanctioned dispute reso-lution system. However, particular systems may define their jurisdiction more narrowly. Within the UK a 'grievance hierarchy' has emerged in which the notion of complaints has become synonymous with less serious, voiced griev-ances, and the legal claim associated with more serious cases. Within the NHS, what is seen as constituting a valid complaint within formal systems depends on the service being complained about. Separate systems operate depending on the location of the treatment, the type of health care worker responsible for the poor care being alleged and the severity of the grievance. Moreover, while the hospital sector has a history of allowing a complaint about any aspect of their service to be heard in their formal complaints systems, the primary care sector has traditionally operated much tighter jurisdictional control over what constitutes a complaint.[18] Central statistics on the incidence of formal complaints about the NHS show that those who pursue their grievances through formal procedures tend to focus on particular NHS services.

The total number of formal complaints about the NHS increased sharply between 1999–2000 and 2000–1 by 11 per cent to 95,994. This increase is set against the overall downward trend reported in the years since a new com-plaints procedure was implemented in April 1996 (DoH 2002). Hospital and community services feature particularly prominently in statistics about formal complaints. They received 94 per cent of the total number of complaints in 2000–1.[19] When these statistics are analysed by profession it is clear that the largest proportion are directed at medical and surgical practitioners (46 per cent) followed by nursing, midwifery and health visiting (20 per cent), and the administrative staff (9 per cent).[20] Significantly, the proportion of complaints about medical and surgical professionals has risen steadily from 38 per cent of the total in 1996–7 to 46 per cent in 2000–1. Research by Mulcahy (2000) suggests medical and surgical professionals in the hospital sector do not all have the same exposure to formal complaints. Table 4.1 shows the mean num-ber of complaints and allegations received by consultants in her sample during their careers.

Table 4.1   The mean number of complaints and allegations received by consultants in different specialties during their careers

Specialty	Mean number of complaints in career	Mean number of allegations in career
Obstetrics and gynaecology	4.5	4.5
Orthopaedics	8.1	4.5
General medicine	3.4	3.6
General surgery	5.1	2.5
Paediatrics	1.9	1.9
Mental illness	2.7	1.8
Geriatrics	2.1	1.7
Dermatology	2.4	1.7
Psychiatry	1.5	1.4
Anaesthetics	1.1	1.0
Haematology	0.8	0.8
Radiology	0.8	0.8
Histopathology	0.3	0.4
All consultants	**2.1**	**1.9**

Source: Mulcahy 2000.

These data need to be contextualized. In particular, it is important to balance them against data on the amount of activity within each of the specialties as the risk of being complained about is more accurately seen in the context of the number of complaints per patient episode. A finding that consultants in obstetrics and gynaecology receive more complaints than many other specialties, for instance, will be of little use if attention is not also drawn to the fact that obstetrics and gynaecology departments also see a higher number of patients than other specialties.

The task of comparing patient contacts with the number of complaints is not an easy one. Although the methods used by Mulcahy are a little crude they do provide an indication of how the data presented on complaints can be contextualized in this way.[21] Data showing consultant activity and specialty by complaints in her study are shown in Table 4.2.

It is clear from the data on consultant activity by specialty that certain features of the four specialties with the lowest number of patient contacts per complaint are shared. Orthopaedics, psychiatry, geriatrics and mental illness are all specialties involving clients with low social status who are likely to feel disempowered by their condition and more likely than other patients to experience discrimination. Conversely, specialists in obstetrics and gynaecology, general surgery and haematology have the highest number of patient contacts per complaint. One reason why general surgeons and haematologists do not receive large numbers of complaints is that, despite a high patient

Table 4.2 Consultant activity and specialty by complaints in the sample

Specialty	No. of complaints	% Complaints (n = 204)	Activity	% Activity (n = 2108059)	No. of patient contacts per complaint
General medicine	34	16.7	207501	9.8	6103
Orthopaedics	25	12.2	23140	11.0	926
Paediatrics	17	8.3	106217	5.0	6248
Psychiatry	19	9.3	19509	0.9	1027
Obstetrics and gynaecology	15	7.3	281089	13.3	18739
Mental illness	13	6.4	61025	2.9	4694
General surgery	11	5.4	206231	9.8	18748
Dermatology	8	3.9	79528	3.8	9941
Geriatrics	6	2.9	29530	1.4	4922
Haematology	2	1.0	56928	2.8	48464

Source: Mulcahy 2000.

throughput, contact with patients in these specialties is increasingly limited. The fact that obstetricians, gynaecologists and general surgeons were within this group is fascinating, given that they are among the consultants most likely to have a legal claim made against them. A possible explanation is that the consequences of error are so great that dissatisfied patients are much more likely to pursue their grievance in law. This explanation has also been put forward in relation to anaesthetics.

It is also apparent from Mulcahy's (2000) study that certain specialties are more likely than others to attract particular types of allegation and these data aid further analysis of complaining dynamics. Figure 4.2 shows the distribution of complaints according to the three main categories of allegation. Much of these data reflects the type of work undertaken by particular disciplines. Specialties such as histopathology and radiology, which are involved in diagnosis rather than treatment, predictably did not receive a high level of allegations about treatment. Similarly, specialties such as radiology and histopathology which involve a strong diagnostic element featured prominently in this cluster of allegations. Comparisons between specialty ranking in the three categories also suggests some interesting trends. Specialities such as general surgery and orthopaedics did not feature prominently in allegations about treatment problems, tests or diagnosis, but they do feature prominently in complaints about communication and attitude.[22]

Other research has confirmed that certain types of grievance are also less likely than others to be voiced. Mulcahy and Tritter (1998) found that grievances relating to management issues are less likely to emerge as a formal

Communication and attitude	Treatment problems (other than surgery)	Tests and diagnosis
HIGH Dermatology (50%) Orthopaedics (44%) General surgery (40%) Radiology (36%) Haematology (33%) Obstetrics and gynaecology (28%)	**HIGH** Anaesthetics (34%) General medicine (30%) Psychiatry (30%) Geriatrics (26%) Mental illness (23%) Paediatrics (23%)	**HIGH** Radiology (50%) Histopathology (40%) Paediatrics (31%) Haematology (25%) General medicine (22%) Psychiatry (18%)
Sample as a whole 26%	**Sample as a whole 18%**	**Sample as a whole 16%**
Paediatrics (25%) Anaesthetics (25%) Geriatrics (21%) Histopathology (20%) Psychiatry (16%) Mental illness (14%) General medicine (14%)	Dermatology (15%) Obstetrics and gynaecology (15%) Haematology (8%) Orthopaedics (4%) General surgery (3%)	Mental illness (14%) Anaesthetics (13%) Dermatology (8%) Obstetrics and gynaecology (7%) Orthopaedics (7%) Geriatrics (5%) General surgery (3%)
LOW	**LOW**	**LOW**

Figure 4.2 The correlation between the most popular allegations and specialty[23]

Source: DoH. Figures are an amalgamation of Finished Consultant Episode, Outpatient Referrals and Consultant Initiated Attendances for Oxford Region, 1993–4.

complaint. Other studies have highlighted the difficulties that patients face in making complaints about technical aspects of care and suggest that complainants prefer to focus on aspects of care over which they can claim knowledge, such as hotel services (Lloyd-Bostock and Mulcahy 1994). Reflecting on years of experience as a complaints manager in the NHS, Truelove (1985: 230) argues that some of the most difficult complaints to deal with are those from 'reluctant complainers' because the complaint may be understated and the temptation may be 'to respond soothingly without properly examining causes for valid dissatisfaction'.

Amongst those doctors interviewed in Mulcahy's study there was little acceptance that the nature of doctor-patient communication was a genuine issue. Most who discussed it felt that they knew how to communicate effectively but were hardly ever given the opportunity in a public health care system. In the words of one consultant cited in the study: 'Communicating well is an expensive luxury. I have never yet had a complaint from one of my private patients because in private practice I have the time to handle all aspects of a case. You can see a complaint coming, so you make a mental note and go the full distance in sorting their dissatisfaction out' (Mulcahy 2000: 99).

For the majority of consultants in the study, technical failure was the only justification for holding doctors to account. Those interviewed were frustrated because, in their view, the use of good communication skills could actually hide the provision of poor care. One argued: 'When you know that something has gone wrong, that's when you pull out all the stops and over-compensate by listening to the patient and making them feel that you really care. When you have a potential lawsuit, good communication may be the only way to protect yourself' (Mulcahy 2000: 102). For this cluster there was an injustice in judging doctors by their ability to interact well rather than by more technical aspects of clinical competence. This viewpoint assumes reliance on a bio-medical model of competence rather than an holistic one but was popular among consultants.

Others viewed the problem from a different perspective and took the high incidence of communication complaints as a deeper and more serious malaise. Almost half the interviewees expressed concerns about what communication issues said about the current state of the doctor-patient relationship and the various ways in which it had moved from the professional ideal. As one consultant argued:

> People look at systems which are their specialty but medicine is an art. We have lost our basic skill; our ability to communicate. We have no choice – GPs are rushed, consultants are rushed. Patients are treated as a body, a disease. It's all about technique these days. It may be because it is a free system – a conveyor belt. It makes us scientific but we lose our humanity.
>
> (Mulcahy 2000: 104)

When it comes to consideration of the type of voiced grievances processed by the legal system it becomes clear that the notion of 'claim' is defined even more restrictively. Not all voiced grievances or formal complaints are capable of being transformed into legal claims. This is because the law does not com-pensate claimants for every harm or disappointment. In their determination of what constitutes a 'legitimate' cause of action, lawyers and legislators delineate between the types of harm which are considered worthy of compen-sation or punishment and those which are not. The overt purpose of these categories is that they reflect political decisions about what it is morally acceptable and economically viable for society to compensate and who should be held to account. They are not set in stone but major changes, or additions to, established categories are rare and slow to be recognized.[24] Use has been made of a host of legal doctrines in attempts by patients to hold doctors to account for mishaps including the law of murder, the tort of trespass, breach of contract, judicial review of administrative action and battery. But by far the most significant device to be used to challenge doctors' decisions and treatment has been the medical negligence action. For the purposes of this book it also provides an apt case study of how the medical profession has been insulated from challenge by another elite profession.

The modern law of medical negligence operates on two principles. These are that the patient must agree to treatment and that the treatment must be carried out with proper skill by the doctors involved. To be successful in bringing an action a claimant must establish five things: the existence of a duty of reasonable care; that a breach of that duty has occurred through substandard care; that this has resulted in injury; that the injury suffered is not too remote from events; and that the claimant has suffered as a consequence. The doctor is not meant to be a miracle worker. Adverse outcomes consistent with what might be considered a 'normal' risk must be borne by the patient although in reality distinguishing between accidents and negligence is often difficult (Ham et al. 1988). But what is most relevant in the current context is *how* the modern law of negligence distinguishes between accidents and negligence. Significantly, it holds doctors and other health care professionals liable only for that subset of iatrogenic injury that results from poor care as defined by a 'respectable' school of medical peers. Since medical opinion can vary significantly between different schools of thought and specialists, a doctor's actions or omissions are acceptable in law if they at least follow practices that would not be disapproved of by a body of responsible doctors within the profession. This general principle, established in the seminal case of *Bolam* v. *Friern Hospital Management Committee*,[25] means that negligence cannot be inferred just because another doctor, or body of doctors, would have taken a contrary view.

There is something of an irony in the shift towards peer review in the judicial consideration of modern claims. The dominant assumption prior to the rise of scientific method in the modern world was that of medical specificity. It was assumed that different people responded to the same treatments in different ways. This meant that medical malpractice actions were unsupportable because there were few objective standards by which to judge practice. Ironically then, it was the growing importance of science which gave doctors social, economic and professional power but which also made them more vulnerable to criticism because of the new belief in objective standards. Interestingly, in its early incarnations, the English common law also failed to make such a clear link between grievances, fault and compensation. It preferred instead to rely on the principle of strict liability in protecting the interests of those who had suffered damage caused by the act or omission of another. In time, however, wrongfulness in a moral sense has come to play a key role in the law of medical negligence and elsewhere.[26] The philosophical foundation of this approach is that the right to damages should depend on showing that the defendant is culpable rather than just being causally responsible. But, in assessing what the defendant deserves in medical negligence cases the approach of common law jurisdictions has been to look at how other doctors behave rather than the motivation of individuals. So, in fact, the use of this objective test may tell us nothing about the moral culpability of the defendant (Merry and McCall Smith 2001). It also fails to tell us anything of the systemic errors which have led to an injury.

Concern has been expressed that because the standard of care is judged by reference to the opinion of other doctors, the court transfers responsibility for determining whether there has been negligence back to the profession itself, represented in court by expert witnesses. For this reason the medical negligence action could be viewed as a form of self-regulation. The courts retain the right to decide between competing arguments about established professional practice but, in practice, the number of cases in which the courts exercise this power is tiny. Thus, the medical profession not only offers evidence of good practice (a factual matter) but also determines what doctors ought to do (a legal matter) (Kennedy and Grubb 2000). It is clear that in adopting and continuing to reinforce the relatively undemanding requirements of the *Bolam* test, English law has endorsed medical autonomy to a much greater extent than other comparable systems and the approach has been strongly criticized in other common law jurisdictions.[27] It is noticeable that the courts in other jurisdictions have placed greater emphasis on the standard of care a *patient would expect to receive*. Arguing from an Australian perspective it has been suggested that the English approach is best understood as a hangover from the Victorian age in which paternalism and a hierarchical class-based society prevailed. Teff (1994) has argued, somewhat ironically, that, if anything, English law has remained more sympathetic to the doctor-centred approach to the provision of health care than the profession itself. He argues that this has resulted in the English courts condoning diagnostic practices and methods of treatment which may have only a modicum of acceptance within the medical profession. Empirical research has demonstrated that the high evidential burden placed on claimants makes the acquisition of compensation unlikely. The problems are such that Lord Woolf devoted a whole chapter to these cases in his groundbreaking review of the civil justice system and referred to the system under review as a 'battleground in which no rules apply' (Lord Chancellor's Department 1996). Figure 4.3, taken from Mulcahy et al.'s (1999) evaluation of the DoH's medical negligence mediation pilot scheme, shows that in the subset of cases handled in such a system only a small proportion of claimants succeed. Their review of just under 4000 closed claims files in two health regions found that less than only 0.4 per cent of cases in the former Anglian region proceeded to trial and only 1 per cent in the former Yorkshire region. Between 70 and 78 per cent of cases were abandoned before formal legal proceedings had even been issued.

In their study of the connection between medical mishaps and claims, Lindgren et al. (1991) found that only 17 per cent of adverse outcomes came about as a result of negligence which would be recognized by the courts. This compares with 28 per cent in the Harvard Medical Malpractice Study (Leape et al. 1991). In part the weak link between these phenomena can be explained

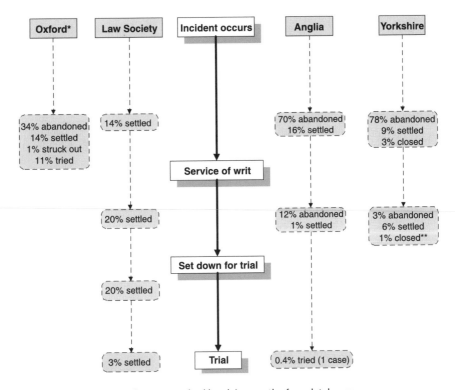

Figure 4.3   Summary of stages reached by claims on the four databases
* No stage identified
** Classified in the database as closed, completed, won
Source: Mulcahy et al. 1999.

by reference to the severity of harm. In the Harvard study, in more than 70 per cent of cases, the injuries involved led to minimal or moderate disability of less than six months' duration and were unlikely to have attracted significant damages. Similarly, Hiatt et al. (1989) found that 70 per cent of instances in which there was evidence of an adverse event led to only slight or short-term injury and Schimmel's study (1964) found that only 20 per cent of iatrogenic injuries to hospital patients were serious or fatal.[28]

Debate about alternative ways of compensating victims of medical mishap has identified the importance of questioning the function of particular grievance systems. In existing schemes for handling claims the burden of proof is high and access to the courts is restricted by cost. As a rationing system which is designed to protect NHS resources the system works well. But it is important to recognize that grievance systems have a number of other goals. Not all of these are compatible. They can be used for early identification and management of risk; as managerial tools in the assessment of quality; as instigators of disciplinary action; as an opportunity to improve the reputation of a Trust or practice; as a formal mechanism for patients to discover more about the care they received; or as a way to resolve disputes. A system that aims to limit the financial liability of a Trust by early suppression of dissatisfaction may not, for example, serve to publicize bad practice or encourage a full disclosure of mistakes which have been made.

Allsop and Mulcahy (2000) have identified two main models for handling information about adverse events, complaints and claims. These can be labelled the 'discrete case' approach and the 'public interest' approach. They are ideal types and in reality there are many hybrid models which exist between the two extremes represented by them. Table 4.3 identifies examples of existing systems which fit into each category.

In the UK, the current system of clinical negligence is a good example of a procedure which individualizes blame. Until recently, mechanisms for complaint handling also tended towards the fault-based model and those operated by professional bodies – such as the GMC, General Dental Council and United Kingdom Central Council for Nursing, Midwifery and Health Visiting (UKCC) – still do. However, the introduction of a new NHS complaints procedure from April 1996 began to place more emphasis on responding to the needs of disputants, the aftermath of complaints and the lessons which could be learned from them. Moreover, the GMC has recently introduced a new layer to its complaint procedures that is rehabilitative and designed to help doctors improve their performance before referring them to more formal disciplinary

Table 4.3   Models for managing information about adverse events, complaints and claims

Discrete case	Hybrid systems	Public interest
Civil justice system	NHS complaints system	**(A) National learning**
United Kingdom Central Council for Nursing, Midwifery and Health Visiting (UKCC)	Health Services Commissioner (HSC) Mediation pilot scheme	Commission for Health Audit and Inspection (CHAI) Patient Safety Agency
General Medical Council		Council of Health Regulators
NHS disciplinary procedures		**(B) Local learning** Risk management
Arbitration		Quality management
		Clinical and medical audit
		Patient satisfaction surveys

processes. In introducing its five-year reaccreditation scheme, the GMC is accepting responsibility for generic quality standards instead of focusing solely on the relatively tiny number of doctors found guilty of professional misconduct each year.

The discrete case approach individualizes grievance resolution and tends to adopt a fault-based standard. Its aim is to identify 'bad apples' responsible for poor performance and punish them. The main feature of such an approach is that it is *reactive* to those who make complaints or claims. It *individualizes* blame by placing the emphasis on investigating the activities of individual actors within the NHS. Individuals within the organization rather than the organization itself will be held responsible. As a result the organization can distance itself from culpability. According to this model, action can only be taken when someone has acted outside the powers allocated to them or been found not to have performed to an acceptable standard. This has the effect of narrowing the scope of what can be complained about. Three other features distinguish this approach. Fault finding is likely to be based on lengthy investigations because the reputations and livelihood of individuals are at stake. Access to appeal structures is limited because of the intensity of investigation, resulting cost and burden of evidence required. Finally, cases that are substantiated are seen as *discrete acts* of poor performance. The discrete case approach is more likely to polarize the positions of the parties because the management of the dispute personalizes blame by investigating the actions of the person blamed. As a result defensiveness becomes an inevitable feature of such systems.

By way of contrast the public interest model has been described as one which places emphasis on what can be learnt from adverse events, complaints and claims. The system is proactive and can lead to dissatisfaction being sought out and complaints encouraged (Cabinet Office Service First Unit 1999). Methods of investigation aim to be pervasive and to involve a wide range of individuals and systems. Emphasis is placed on systemic failures as well as individual responsibility. Architects of such systems argue that adversarial situations are avoided and resolution and redress are used as a way of maintaining relationships and organizational loyalty. The introduction of the clinical negligence mediation pilot scheme is an example of this approach. Although issues of fault and individual blame still remained important in the mediations conducted, some of the remedies supplied by Trusts to injured patients reflected a recognition that it was important for claimants to understand how their claim had changed the way care is delivered. The introduction of a requirement that certain key actors see the reports of IRPs at the final stage of the 1996 complaints procedure also indicated a shift away from a purely fault-based model, as does the heightened expectations in the 1996 system that information about complaints will be fed into quality management systems. In addition, no-fault compensation schemes exist in a number of other jurisdictions which have abandoned the rule that an injured patient has to show that someone was negligent in order to obtain compensation. Based on a distributive justice model the social need to compensate those with disabilities from government funds is given precedence over the need to punish those who are responsible for the harm or make an example of them. There are many different types of scheme but they all attempt to spread the losses for medical accidents over entire populations of consumers of medical services and taxpayers (see further Bovbjerg et al. 1997; Ridgway 1999; Whetten-Goldstein et al. 1999; Erichsen 2001; Studdert and Brennan 2001).[29] UK policy makers have flirted with the idea of introducing no-fault compensation in the past, and at the time of writing are once again considering this option. This alone is evidence of the ways in which debate about the aims and functions of grievance systems are in a constant state of flux which reflect changing notions of the ideas of the accountability of the medical profession and the state's responsibility to victims of medical mishap.

Conclusion

This chapter set out to explore how medical mishaps, dissatisfaction with health care, complaints and medical negligence claims are conceptualized and how the links between them are best understood. It has become clear during the course of this analysis that none of these phenomena could be said to be naturally occurring. Each term reflects a fluid quality which says more about the cultural and political context in which we try to understand it than it does about the activity which researchers have attempted to explain. Throughout the chapter it has become apparent that experts, and particularly medical experts, retain considerable power over defining what is deviant, be it a medical mishap, complaint or legal claim. Perhaps what is most striking about the work discussed here is that while the rising incidence of complaints and claims is seen as a crisis by some, others, employing the discourse of rights, could justifiably see it in positive terms. The research visited here actually suggests that the rate of complaints remains modest when compared to the number of grievances. Studies reviewed in this chapter suggest that disputes may be relatively uncommon when compared against a baseline of perceived injurious experiences and that western societies are uncontentious and even passive. In view of the data presented it could even be argued that there is too little conflict surfacing in society and that too few wrongs are perceived, pursued and remedied. According to this view, conflict and disputes are seen as a healthy indication of the accessibility of law and legal systems. This view is in stark contrast to those who have fuelled fears of a medical litigation crisis. It is certainly interesting to reflect how powerful the image has become, among doctors, of law and the courts as meddlesome intruders in medical affairs. It is true that law is increasingly being invoked to determine and limit the power of doctors, but when one looks more closely at how the standard in medical negligence cases is determined it is clear that the English courts have been more than content to let medical perceptions of patient welfare prevail. It may be that, because most doctors have but a hazy knowledge of law, the complaints and claims become a symbol of the limits of medical authority, even if statistically they are but a phantom menace.

Notes

1 So, for instance, medical negligence and malpractice are terms which are used by lawyers and have developed very precise legal meanings.
2 This is a higher standard than that imposed by the courts where only one expert is usually required per litigant. Andrews et al.'s particular critique is aimed at the Harvard study which is discussed throughout this chapter. I believe that the comments also have a more general applicability.
3 The literature on adverse events in hospital settings is growing by the month. In addition to the research alluded to in the text see: Bates et al. (1998); Petersen and Waddell (1998); Gawande et al. (1999); Krizek (2000); Vincent (1995); Bates (2000); Boreham et al. (2000); Ayuzawa (2001); Beran (2001); Chalcroft (2001); Davis et al. (2001); Higgins (2001); McIlwain (2001); Savage and Armstrong (1990). It should be noted that the same is not true of a primary care setting (but see Sheikh and Hurwitz 2001).
4 In 1964 Schimmel reported that 20 per cent of patients admitted to hospital suffered iatrogenic injury. Steele (1977) found that 36 per cent of patients admitted to hospital suffered an iatrogenic event. More than half of the injuries involved medication. In terms of medical error in an intensive care unit, an average of 1.7 errors per patient per day occurred of which 29 per cent had the potential to result in serious or fatal injury.
5 See, for example, Brook et al. (1973). Andrews et al. (1997) suggest that the reason why other studies have identified a higher incidence of adverse events is that the definitions used in the Harvard study were more restrictive and based on legal-policy models.
6 Thomas and Brennan (2000) found that elderly patients had a particularly high exposure to preventable adverse events relating to drugs, medical procedures and falls. They also tended to experience more permanent injury and death as a result. However, after adjustments were made for the complexity of care and other patient and hospital characteristics, age was not an independent correlate of preventable adverse events. The authors suggest that the difference in the incidence when elderly patients are compared to younger ones is that the former tend to have much more complex treatments and care plans. See also Marcantonio et al. (1999).

7   It was pointed out in *An Organisation with a Memory* (DoH 2000b) that medical mishaps represent a cost in terms of additional hospital days and in the settlement of claims. Considerable staff time is also spent in dealing with the aftermath of medical mishaps and with complaints and claims when they arise. The National Patient Safety Agency was set up in 2001 and will have the responsibility for developing an improved system for reporting, analysing and acting on these phenomena so as to develop systems to prevent them arising in the first place.

8   In this context, I refer only to identification of a medical error. Dissatisfaction may also arise, quite legitimately, with the way in which care was provided.

9   The authors of this study make the point that being in hospital longer enhances situational power as patients in this category are more likely to understand the systems and culture of the organization.

10 The whole relationship between dissatisfaction with specific incidents of medical care and more global ratings of medical care has also been underexplored. Fitzpatrick (1993) has argued that the sole use of global scores may disguise particular instances of dissatisfaction while yielding a high satisfaction score. Despite this, there is some evidence that instruments designed to measure reactions to specific instances of care received are more accurate (Roberts et al. 1983).

11 Clearly the method used to collect data can also have a profound effect on what emerges. For instance, Strasser and Davis (1991) found that close-ended questions on hospital surveys tend to yield positive evaluations while open-ended questions produce negative responses.

12 In response to these concerns, some commentators have attempted to approach dissatisfaction as a multidimensional construct which is not necessarily related to a particular event or circumstance (Roghmann et al. 1979; Fitzpatrick 1991, 1993; Hopkins 1993; Thompson 1993). According to this approach, dissatisfaction is seen as a sentiment which is the product of a complex interaction between patients' perceptions, expectations, their history of care and their emotional state (Locker and Dunt 1978; Linder-Pelz 1982).

13 It was rather depressing to discover that at the time their claim was 'closed' 24 per cent and 22 per cent respectively still wanted to achieve these goals.

14 Eleven of these 13 had been identified by the study as being the subject of an adverse event. For these 11 claiming patients the number of adverse events per patient ranged from 1 to 33 with the mean being just under 10 events per patient.

15 Only two previous empirical studies have looked at the relationship between legal claims and complaints and both suggest that the 'danger' of complaints progressing to claims may have been overstated by policy makers. In their study of hospital complaints in a UK setting, Mulcahy and Lloyd-Bostock (1994) explored the issue of the proportion of complaints which had the potential to become claims. First, they looked at whether the allegations made

might constitute a recognized cause of action. They focused on: whether the complaint related to clinical care; whether an allegation of physical harm had been made; the severity of physical harm alleged; and any attributions of fault and requests for compensation. Second, they looked for any indications that the complainant might want to pursue the complaint further, such as the use of solicitors and other agents and the stage that the complaint reached in the complaints machinery. Their study suggested that, even when cases which fell into all these categories were added together, only 4 per cent of complaints had the potential to 'progress' to legal claims.

The second study, undertaken in an American setting by Jost et al. (1993), made use of the conceptual approach developed by Mulcahy and Lloyd-Bostock in its examination of the possible overlap between complaints to the Ohio State Licensure Board and the tort system. An analysis was undertaken of 200 records of complaints made to the Medical Board, a GMC-like regulatory body that uses complaints to determine whether a doctor should have their professional registration suspended. Two indications of a claim were looked for: suggestions that the complaint was capable of being lodged as a medical negligence action and indications on the file that the complainant had independently filed a malpractice suit. The study found that, in spite of the fact that 16 complainants mentioned contacting an attorney prior to filing the complaint and that 11 threatened a lawsuit, only 2 (1 per cent) complainants actually filed a lawsuit before, or after, making their complaint.

16   Seventy-three per cent of the 240 patients in their 'dissatisfied' sample.

17   *Handling Complaints* (DoH 2001) did not indicate that access to information was a problem but its sample was taken from people who had complained.

18   Until 1994, complaints about primary care had to relate to a breach in the terms of service contract negotiated between the state and the BMA.

19   Ambulance Trusts received 4 per cent and health authorities and primary care Trusts received a total of 3 per cent.

20   The category 'other' accounts for a further 11 per cent.

21   Activity in hospitals is recorded in a number of different ways and for a variety of different purposes. When a patient first enters hospital they will be given a READ code which provides a narrative description of their condition from which a certain level of activity might be predicted. Thereafter they are categorized by an ICD code, a detailed diagnosis code which reflects the type of procedures undertaken. The only datasets which record the specific activity of consultants appear to be Finished Consultants Episodes (FCEs), Referral Attendances to consultants and Consultant Initiated Attendances. These three sets of figures were used as a broad indicator of the number of patients consultants in each specialty can be expected to come into contact with each year. However, there are difficulties in using these figures as a yardstick against which to judge activity. Only one episode of any kind is recorded per patient treatment, so that in procedures where more than one consultant is concerned

with the care, only one of them will have the FCE recorded. Thus, consultants who facilitate the making of decisions about diagnosis and treatment, such as laboratory-based specialties and haematology, are hardly represented at all. Moreover, one very large specialty, anaesthetics, appears to be extremely under-represented. Some of these difficulties can be overcome. By using generic categories of specialties it is more probable that teams of consultant activity will be reflected across discrete specialities. For instance, by using the category 'surgical', the work of anaesthetists is captured in the figures. Also, particular emphasis can be placed on comparing levels of activity with complaints in those specialties where these data are more reliable indicators of patient contacts.

22   A handful of consultants argued that colleagues practising in what they labelled 'people specialties', such as psychotherapy, where communicating is an integral part of the treatment being provided, were much less likely to get a complaint because the patient's concerns would be fully explored as part of the process. This suggestion appears to be borne out by the data presented in the figures as communication complaints do not feature prominently in mental illness and psychiatry, although this might also be explained by the fact that patients in such specialities are less empowered than others. However, an endocrinologist also suggested: 'My specialty prompts very few complaints. It involves long-term care plans. It is both fascinating and necessary to get patients involved from the start in drawing up a care plan and setting object-ives. As a result, patients have a high level of understanding, despite the fact that many of the concepts involved are hard to explain. I believe that we do not get complaints because we are in a position to share information'.

23   I was concerned that data on some specialties would not yield reliable figures since the number of consultants representing them in the sample was low and their experience might be atypical. To allow for this, all those specialties which featured responses from at least ten consultants were extracted – this being regarded as the smallest meaningful figure of use in comparing percentages. This method yielded 13 specialties about which it is possible to make more general comments. Of these, dermatology, general medicine, general surgery, mental illness, obstetrics and gynaecology and orthopaedics received more than the mean number of complaints (2.1), geriatrics received the average and anaesthetics, haematology, histopathology, paediatrics, psychiatry and radiology received fewer than average.

24   Current debates about the notion of wrongful birth are a good example of this point. See further the discussions in *McFarlane* v. *Tayside* HB [2000] 2 AC 59; *Rees* v. *Darlington Memorial Hospital* [2002] EWCA Civ 88; *Emeh* v. *Kensington, Chelsea and Westminster AHA* [1985] QB 1012 and the commentaries in Dickens (1990) and Donnelly (1997). In the last few decades debates have also raged about such issues as the legalization of abortion, the termination of life, the treatment of handicapped neonates and genetic engineering.

25 [1957] WLR 586.

26 Despite this, notions of strict liability have begun to replace fault-based negligence in some fields, such as product liability where manufacturers are better able to compensate for harm than individual victims. A similar rationale has been used in cases involving insurers. See, for example, *Nettleship* v. *Weston* [1971] 3 All ER 581.

27 See, for example, *Rogers* v. *Whitaker* [1992] 175 CLR 479.

28 But in 7 per cent of cases the injury was permanent and 14 per cent of patients died as a result of their treatment.

29 Sweden introduced a patient insurance scheme in 1975 as a result of complaints that few victims of medical mishaps were getting compensation because of the difficulties of proving fault and finding experts to support a claim, as well as the expense and delay involved. The Treatment Injury Insurance Scheme introduced in Finland in 1987 provides a similar scheme. A no-fault scheme was introduced in New Zealand in 1971 which covered all disabilities resulting from accidents and not just injuries caused by medical negligence. In the USA, the states of Virginia (1988) and Florida (1989) have introduced schemes covering birth injuries. An important distinction must be made between those schemes that require patients to identify the individual who is responsible for their condition and those that do not. The former have the advantage of being able to make constructive use of the desire of injured patients to obtain redress in a similar way to the clinical negligence system. Adverse outcomes can be attributed to individual doctors and can be used to contribute to quality agendas. The doctors involved can be asked to provide information about the treatment given to the claimant so that the quality of their care can be assessed. They may also be asked to cooperate with reviews of their licence to practise. Those schemes that sever the link between victims and the agents of their injuries must find alternative ways of achieving this objective.

5 Forever amber?

Looking at disputes with doctors from the perspective of the complainant

Introduction

So far in this book the discussion of disputes between doctors and patients has focused on the broader political context in which they take place. By way of contrast the next three chapters focus on a micro-level analysis of the socio-legal dynamics of such disputes. They consider what the parties hope to achieve from their interaction, how they voice their needs and justify their behaviour, and the ways in which individual disputes reflect the broader themes considered in earlier chapters. It is argued that many of the tensions which emerge from stories of complaints and claims are the same as those which have arisen during the course of negotiations between the government, consumer groups and the medical profession about the respective roles of doctors and patients in our society. These grievances and explanations reveal much about the normative frameworks within which all of these actors operate, their expectations of the boundaries of the doctor-patient relationship and the ways in which such boundaries are the subject of constant negotiation.

The accounts which emerge from disputes between doctors and complainants are all forms of impression management involving important and revealing identity work. They are tales of untoward events and circumstances whose function is to exculpate the actor from responsibility or at least mitigate the possibility of negative moral judgements being made of them. Such impression management is achieved through a number of devices in a disputing context but most noticeably through blame and justification (Tedeschi and Reiss 1981). It is clear from the empirical studies discussed in forthcoming chapters that what is debated during these exchanges is what doctors, managers and complainants consider socially acceptable by reference to their own personal values and those of the groups to which they belong. It is argued in this chapter that complaints need to be understood and analysed at two different levels. From a macro perspective they mirror the increasing emphasis in our society on consumerism, individualism and a discourse of rights. The first section of this chapter focuses on this issue. But these disputes also need to be understood at a micro level. Complaints need to be explored as complex everyday social processes in which the debates of the elite are played out. The second section of the chapter focuses on this theme and considers what is at stake for complainants when they voice their grievances. The chapter concludes with a consideration of how the needs of complainants are to be responded to and the extent to which the remedies available in legal systems are inappropriate for many of them.

The broader context

Complaints are a form of consumer activism which reflect wider social changes heralded, among others, by the civil rights movements and second-wave feminism. The incidence of complaints and claims has increased in the past 20 years, an era in which attention was drawn to the ways in which the rights of the socially excluded had been marginalized. During this time, academic debate has centred on how participatory democracy could be achieved as trust in authority was questioned. Changing attitudes have been reflected most obviously in the rise of consumerism in the post-Fordist era. During this time, consumer groups have emerged as a political force demanding improved conditions and rights for the wider population.[1] The intimacy of the doctor-patient relationship, the potential for exploitation and the serious consequences of medical mistakes have been used by many of these groups as justifications for greater regulation of professionals in the interests of consumer choice and autonomy.[2] Consumer activism has expressed itself in a number of ways such as complaints and litigation, political campaigns, persuasion, non-compliance with treatment plans and more obviously through public political debate.[3]

While access to the legitimizing discourse of science has enabled medics to assume excessive social power in defining 'reality' and identifying deviance and social disorder,[4] consumer groups have argued that a scientific knowledge base is not the only one through which health and illness can be understood. Patients have argued that experience of health care gives the patient a unique perspective on what constitutes appropriate treatment and that this should be taken more seriously in diagnosis and treatment decisions. They have argued that distinctions between doctors and patients made on the basis of a chasm between lay and medical knowledge are inappropriate. Not only has it been argued that not all medical issues are so complex that they cannot be understood by the laity, but patients have also argued that their experience of medical conditions represents an alternative way of knowing (see e.g. Oakley 1980). The report of the Bristol Inquiry, prompted by whistle-blowers and complainants, identified a general need to return to shared decision making and open communication between doctors and patients as a priority. In the words of its authors:

> The contrast which we seek to draw is between a system in which interaction with patients becomes routed through a complaints system, such that comments become complaints, even if they did not begin as such, and a system which allows multiple opportunities for communication between the hospital and those it serves. The future lies in the latter.
>
> (Bristol Inquiry 2001, para. 50)

The state has come to accept the increasing importance of the consumer voice in the provision of health care. Not only do such policies receive favour with the electorate, they also reflect a recognition by policy makers that managers cannot always represent the views of patients when dealing with the medical profession. The formation of state-funded CHCs in 1974 did much to help strengthen the consumer voice in policy making, although they continued to be unpopular with politicians as many adopted a much more radical stance than was originally anticipated. The privatization and contracting out initiatives of the Thatcher governments and others since has further encouraged consumer activism. New notions of accountability and public service came about as a result of the Next Steps programme, the creation of internal markets, the *Citizen's Charter* and the publication of data about NHS performance indicators (Cabinet Office 1988). These have all aimed to increase efficiency and provide greater accountability to consumers at the level of service delivery through complaints and other mechanisms.[5] This new focus on consumerism has also led to increased enthusiasm to expand and develop the monitoring of consumer views (Longley 1993). For the more cynical, this emphasis on complaints has allowed the rhetoric of consumerism to support moves towards a compliance culture. In turn, this has facilitated an increased vigilance of professionals by the state under the guise of protection and promotion of service users. In this sense the emphasis on consumerism is inextricably linked to the emergence of managerialism in the NHS (Nettleton and Harding 1994).

Consumer activists have consistently argued for models of regulation which favour their interests. In this 'grass roots' approach the emphasis is on empowering users of services by allowing them to maintain control over decision making (see e.g. National Consumer Council 1994, 1999). The emphasis placed on patient power is synonymous with a legal discourse which privileges the individual as the bearer of a right to autonomy and self-determination. The language of law assumes that legal rights confer dignity and respect by recognizing the claims of the abused. One of the reasons why commentators have argued that law has become the greatest threat to medicine in our society is that the rhetoric of law is one which places emphasis on the empowerment and equality of individuals rather than placing them in a knowledge hierarchy. In a health context these changes are reflected in the ways in which medical harm came to be viewed through the lens of individual rights. This trend was particularly noticeable in the decisions of the courts in medical negligence cases where notions of informed consent and duties of disclosure have come to be discussed more seriously. The British judiciary has displayed a slightly more reticent approach to patient autonomy than its counterparts in other jurisdictions, but even they have not been able to escape exposure to such debates or the need to discuss the issues raised.

The perspectives of particular complainants

These wider changes in society have given complaining and making a legal claim more legitimacy than was previously the case, but the costs to individuals in the voicing of a grievance remain considerable. It has been argued in earlier chapters that complaining and claiming is an atypical response to dissatisfaction and the emergence of a grievance. If this proposition is true, it makes those who voice their grievances of particular interest and calls into doubt the popular image of compensation-hungry patients. In their discussion of the tenacity demonstrated by complainants in a health care setting Mulcahy et al. (1996a) argue that far from being characterized as excessively adversarial, complainants often felt impotent when voicing their dissatisfaction and helpless in the face of professional knowledge and status. In the eyes of the complainants interviewed, complaint making required determination, stamina and moral courage. Mulcahy et al. conclude that many complainants voiced their grievances *despite* their feelings that it would not have much impact (Mulcahy et al. 1996a; see also NHSE 1994). What motivates patients and their relatives to step out of role and challenge the appropriateness of what they have been told and had done to them? What do they seek to achieve? How do they go about challenging the actions of expert workers? How do they validate their accounts and justify their actions? What stories do they tell of the effect of medical care upon them?

The characteristics of complaints and complainants

Unlike legal claims, complaints are not restricted to patients or the parents of a minor patient. In their study of hospital complaints Lloyd-Bostock and Mulcahy (1994) found that almost half of the 399 records they looked at concerned the experience of someone other than a complainant, usually a relative. Of those complaining on behalf of another, 68 per cent were performing a caring or visiting role for the patient. In 113 (53 per cent) of cases patients had died or were unable to complain on their own behalf because they were a child, very ill or elderly. In Allsop's (1994) study of primary care complaints, 85 per cent of complaints were made on behalf of others for similar reasons. Lloyd-Bostock and Mulcahy (1994) have argued that those described as making complaints on behalf of others are often expressing their own dissatisfaction rather than being seen as a proxy or agent. In support of this finding they found instances in which the complaint was being made against the patient's wishes.

Complaints do not follow a rigid imposed order as legal claims or responses to surveys may do. Studies have found that it is not always obvious from the letter of complaint what it is that the complainant seeks. In their analysis of 342 letters of complaint, Lloyd-Bostock and Mulcahy (1994) found that in 98 cases (29 per cent) the complainant made no statement at all about what they wanted to happen as a result of their complaint and a further 73 letters (21 per cent) contained only vague requests such as a desire that the hospital 'resolve the matter' or 'take some action':

> a number of statements of the substance of the complaint included a general statement, such as 'the whole stay was a misery' or 'the nurses are uncaring'. In these cases, more specific allegations (e.g., that the patient was left in a wet bed for several hours), rather than being in themselves the substance of the complaint, became illustrations of a more general or global complaint.
>
> (Lloyd-Bostock and Mulcahy 1994: 135)

Mulcahy and Tritter's (1998) study of patients suggested that those who chose to voice their grievance were often reluctant to label their activity as complaining. Of the 326 respondents they interviewed who had voiced a grievance, only 134 (41 per cent) classified their activity in this way. These data reflect a sensitivity to the difficulties in applying the label of complaint and a potential mismatch between the expectations of service users and the architects of complaints procedures. The difficulty of applying labels to such activity is reported by one interviewee who said: 'No, I wasn't making a complaint. If I had wanted to make a complaint I would have gone to the boss of the health authority and not the individual GP. Mind you, I expect he [the GP] went home and told his wife that some silly bugger had been complaining about him today' (p. 842).

Allegations

Complainants make a wide variety of allegations in formal complaints which range from concerns about the size of a boiled egg during a hospital stay to claims about the mismanagement of birth leading to a serious disability. The DoH has never collected data on the type of allegations made in complaints, although it has always collated statistics on whether complaints in the hospital sector are wholly clinical, partly clinical or have no clinical element.[6] Although a distinction between clinical and non-clinical complaints was of interest in the pre-1996 procedure because it determined which type of investigation and appeals procedure should be used, it is of less use in trying to determine the focus of complaints because the division between what constitutes a clinical or non-clinical allegation is not always as clear as might be anticipated.[7] Criticism of poor communication skills might for instance touch upon notions of informed consent or may involve rudeness. Empirical studies have also indicated that allegations vary according to the service being complained about. These variations are undoubtedly a reflection of the type of allegations which historically could be 'heard' in the different procedures that operated in the primary and secondary care sectors.[8]

Problems have arisen in attempts to characterize complaints by allegations. In their content analysis of complaint letters and follow-up interviews with the authors of the letters, Lloyd-Bostock and Mulcahy (1994) have drawn attention to the ways in which formal letters of complaint can fail to capture the nature of the grievance felt. During the course of interviews with complainants they found that complainants' concerns often went way beyond the worries expressed in their letters. Significantly, complainants who had written with criticisms of administrative or 'hotel' services often expressed dissatisfaction with aspects of the medical care received when interviewed face to face. When probed about why they had limited their written account, interviewees expressed a lack of confidence in undermining the validity of medical decision making and were worried that they were less likely to be believed if they challenged a doctor. For this group, the protest was important even if it was incomplete in formal terms. These data suggest that complainants are only too aware of traditional expectations of how patients and others carry out their sick role. They also hint at the fact that the process of responding to a complaint may prove frustrating to both sides as a result of underlying issues not being aired.

Perhaps most significantly for the present study, a comparison of doctors' and patients' views on the key issues raised by complaints suggests that they place emphasis on different aspects of the dispute between them. When she compared the data she collected from hospital consultants with that collected in an earlier study of hospital complainants which used the same allegation codes, Mulcahy (2000) found that data from a one-year cohort of complainants focused on communication and attitude problems (37 per cent), general care of the patient (12 per cent) and waiting times (22 per cent). Complainants identified fewer problems relating to treatment (15 per cent), tests and diagnosis (9 per cent) and problems with surgery (2 per cent).[9] In contrast, consultants focused their discussions of the allegations contained in complaints on problems relating to surgery (11 per cent) and less often on communication issues (25 per cent) than was the case in the other dataset. While the findings are far from conclusive as the two studies focused on different but overlapping samples,[10] it is suggested that the difference may reflect a tendency on the part of doctors to concentrate on technical aspects of care while patients are more likely to emphasize experiential aspects or concerns about the dignity and respect afforded them. Discussing similar findings in her research on complaints in the primary care sector, Allsop (1994: 158) has concluded:

> Generalising from this case study of 110 cases, an obvious point is that the parties to such disputes make their complaints from differing perspectives. They interpret what has occurred from the point of view of their own experiences, interests, knowledge and their ideas about their obligations and responsibilities for handling illness.[11]

I have argued elsewhere that communication allegations provide a particularly startling example of the differing perspectives from which doctors and patients approach care (Mulcahy 2000). The high incidence of complaints relating to communication does not necessarily result from inattentiveness or insensitivity but from a more fundamental disagreement about the nature of illness. In a similar vein, Williams and Popay (1994) have suggested that the differences between the ways in which professionals and the laity represent matters of health and illness have clearly demonstrated that lay beliefs about illness are often quite distinctive in form and content from those held by doctors. It has been argued that rather than representing a shared reality between doctor and patient, illness represents two distinct realities or a systematic distortion of meanings (MacIntyre and Oldman 1977; Blaxter 1983; Cornwall 1984; Toombs 1992; Arksey 1994). The patient and doctor are motivated to attend to different aspects of a 'shared' experience. Because each gives it meaning in a qualitatively distinct manner, communication is not always possible and is at the very least distorted. This makes it particularly difficult for the parties to construct a world of shared meaning and for managers and administrators to mediate between these two perspectives. In Toombs' words:

> The physician is trained to perceive illness essentially as a collection of physical signs and symptoms which define a particular disease state. He or she thematizes the illness as being a particular case of 'multiple sclerosis', 'diabetes', 'peptic ulcer', and so forth. The patient, however, focuses on a different 'reality'. One does not 'see' one's own illness primarily as a disease process. Rather one experiences it essentially in terms of its effects upon everyday life.
>
> (1992: 11)

The more scientific narratives used by doctors have to be learnt during the process of training to become a medic. Toombs (1992) suggests that in the practice of a profession certain 'habits of mind' develop that provide a horizon of meaning by means of which reality is interpreted and reflects the culture of a profession. Most significantly, society affords a status to medical discourse which has never been enjoyed by patients. The social and political status given to doctors and science in our society means that greater status and credibility is assigned to medical accounts of care. Looking at how this is reflected in the patient encounter, Mishler (1984) noted that doctors tend to control the form and content of interviews by defining what is considered relevant. He argues that in medical interviews the voice of the lifeworld tends to be seen as not medically relevant and is typically suppressed. Similarly, in her study of how hospital consultants interpreted allegations made in complaints, Mulcahy (2000) found that doctors focused on what complaints revealed, or failed to reveal, about technical expertise. Viewed in this way the lay challenges contained in complaints do not relate to the aesthetics of discourse but are more accurately seen as a political challenge to the status of scientific knowledge, and reflect a rupture in the compact between state, profession and patient.

The impact of medical mishaps, dissatisfaction and grievances

It is also important to place complainants' accounts in the context of the impact that their complaint, and the circumstances which led to it, has had on their lives. An appreciation of the effects of such events is helpful in understanding motivations to complain, the type of remedies sought and general thresholds of tolerance. The damage described by complainants may be physical, mental, financial or involve a loss of personhood and humanity.[12] Empirical studies demonstrate that voiced grievances about medical care frequently make mention of the physical symptoms of an alleged mistake or episode of poor care and use these as a form of evidence for the allegations made. In their study, Lloyd-Bostock and Mulcahy (1994) found that 38 per cent (150) of letters from complainants alleged that some form of physical harm had been caused. In 19 of these cases a form of permanent harm such as long-term loss of function was alleged and 30 involved a form of temporary but major harm such as burns and delays in diagnosis. Vincent et al. (1993) found, among their sample of 101 potential complainants and claimants, that 74 per cent of patients rated the overall effect on their lives as severe or very severe and 35 per cent experienced severe financial difficulties. They found that increased pain, injuries to an organ, perforation, wound infections and nerve damage accounted for most of the injuries mentioned. They judged the overall effect of alleged negligence to be considerable, leading to increased pain or decreased mobility (30 per cent) and psychological trauma (16 per cent). On average the medical accident patients they surveyed after 16 months had levels of pain comparable to those of unmedicated patients recovering from surgery.

There is also considerable potential for medical accidents and grievances to cause emotional trauma, in fact complaints commonly reflect the fact that patients and their relatives are experiencing some sort of emotional hurt. Ennis and Vincent (1994) argue that grievances about medical error are worse than other mishaps in society because patients and their relatives believe themselves to have been injured by people who they assumed to be dedicated to helping them. Researchers have found that mishaps can lead to anger, distress, pain and disability which in turn may affect employment prospects, financial security, and relationships with family and friends. Symptoms of depression, anxiety, irritability, intrusive memories and sleep disturbance are also common. Vincent et al. (1993) found victims of medical mishap appeared to have much more difficulty adjusting to their medical condition than those with similar injuries which had occurred 'naturally'. Significantly, it would seem that the physical and emotional effects of mishap can be exacerbated if a grievance about the standard of care ensues, and that this can further hinder recovery. Many of the emotional and psychological effects described above are heightened when a patient or their advocate believes that another person caused the problem (Ennis and Vincent 1994). Blaming others can challenge deeply-held views and leave complainants feeling vulnerable and unsure of who they can trust to alleviate their suffering.[13]

Allsop (2001) has argued that particular attention should be paid to death as a motivating factor in making a complaint. Her study found that 47 per cent of complaint letters in a general practice setting related to the death of a patient. The study was not unique in finding that deaths are strongly associated with complaints in this context. Owen's (1991) study of formal complaints against GPs found that a death had occurred in just under one-third of cases (31 per cent). It is to be anticipated that the emotional trauma experienced by complainants in cases relating to death is likely to be particularly intense. In her description of the feelings described in the letters relating to those suffering a bereavement, Allsop draws attention to the common use of words such as 'trust', 'betrayal', 'anger' and 'anguish'. In her comparison of these cases with a cohort of all complaints received by a health authority over ten years she found that complaints relating to a death were much more likely to call for a doctor to be punished, prevented from working or dismissed. But the significance of these cases in the present context goes beyond the intensity of the emotions experienced. Allsop (2001: 1) argues that the making of a complaint can also play a part in the process of mourning. In her words:

> One obvious consequence of a complaint is that the dead person continues to have a social and indeed, legal, existence. For complainants,

the process of bringing a complaint maintains that relationship. A complaint generates activity and interaction between those who are bereaved and a variety of other persons with informal and formal social roles.

In addition to the original event or circumstances complained about, further grievances may emerge which relate to the way the complaint is handled. Sensitive handling of a complaint or claim is so important to complainants that it can be seen as one of the substantive outcomes of settlement or resolution. In their extensive review of the impact of legal claims Ennis and Vincent (1994) argue that the explanation that the patient is given and the support they receive from health care professionals can have a significant and long-lasting effect on their physical and mental well-being. Reflecting on her experience as chair of the Patients Association, Robinson (1999: 246) has argued:

> All of us who did the work were radicalized by it. What impressed me was not just the extent of medical disasters, but also the profound additional damage inflicted when patients and the bereaved failed to get answers and were met with a stone wall of silence or outright lies. Families were stuck like flies in amber, reliving and repeatedly describing the incident they wanted someone to believe.

It is clear that one of the key successes of the DoH's medical negligence mediation pilot scheme was that, in contrast to traditional claims management, it gave claimants the opportunity to participate in the settlement of the dispute.[14] Interviews with claimants demonstrated that not only did they want to have their say but that effective patient-centred face-to-face discussion with the other side also satisfied their need for a form of ritualistic closure of the dispute. Gaining compensation in order to alleviate the effects of injury was important to these interviewees but so too was catharsis, personal explanations and apologies. The additional remedies provided in the cases mediated included full explanations of medical conditions, the rationale for treatment decisions and the likely causes of mistakes; an offer to tour a department with a senior manager in order to see the improvements made as a result of the claim; a new treatment plan at another hospital; a public apology in a press statement; and information about the location of a miscarried foetus' place of burial. In several of the mediations a significant proportion of time was devoted to the presentation of a full explanation of the medical processes which had led to the mishap and these interactions were frequently described as turning points in the resolution process (Mulcahy et al. 1999).[15]

How do complainants construct their account?

It is clear from the arguments made so far that the act of complaining is an emotionally charged event. When complainants voice their grievances they are indicating that they feel damaged in some way. The structure of their accounts also reveals much about their expectations of care, the nature of the doctor-patient relationship and the type of evidence they think it relevant to present when challenging doctors. Their claims to legitimacy and the rhetorical devices they employ uncover much about the boundaries of the doctor-patient relationship and situated power. Allsop (1998) describes the 'universe' of complaint letters as a moral one in which identities are at stake. She suggests that in writing letters complainants seek to protect their own moral identity as patients, carers and complainants. This is because criticizing a doctor is not a safe or familiar activity as many complainants have only a hazy notion of a doctor's formal responsibilities. As a consequence, letters of complaint contain a variety of attempts to demonstrate their complaint-worthiness (Lloyd-Bostock and Mulcahy 1994). Complaint letters are a vehicle for complainants to establish themselves as competent patients and lay carers, and to establish that the failure event was not their fault. This is often done by invoking the doctor's professional responsibilities, referring to past events and the opinion of others, and constructing a positive account of their own part in providing care.

In their study of 399 letters of complaint, Lloyd-Bostock and Mulcahy (1994) found that despite the great variety of complaints, letters fell into a number of clear patterns. All letters stated the matter complained about, in a short sentence or several pages setting out details with times and dates. In addition to detailing the allegations made, letters comprised statements making the implicit or explicit case that the event or circumstance referred to was a valid subject of complaint. Statements in this category often included details of the type and severity of emotional response as well as other ways in which the event or circumstance complained about had affected the complainant's life. Complainants commonly recognized that making a complaint is a hostile act that needed justifying and may invoke a hostile response. As a result, they made efforts to pre-empt the hospital from dismissing the complaint as unjustified, mistaken or trivial. They commonly stressed why a matter which might appear trivial to the hospital had had a more significant impact on them. For example, complainants pointed out that the vulnerable or frail state of the patient magnified the importance of an incident (69 letters), that the consequences could have been far more serious (26 letters) and that the incident indicated a more general problem (23 letters).

Many socio-legal scholars discuss grievances in terms of entitlement and rights but complainants did not use this language. However, this did not stop them making use of the concept of justice and common-sense morality.

Reference to standards of human dignity, politeness, comfort and fairness were common and in some cases were discussed in the context of standards which a professional might be expected to revere such as confidentiality and respect. In her analysis of 58 letters of complaint about GPs in one health authority between 1982 and 1986, Allsop assessed that doctors were labelled as unprofessional in 51 of the letters. At one end of the spectrum, she found that doctors were accused of being 'disinterested' or 'distant' and at the other of being 'cruel', 'threatening' or 'abusive' (2001: 228). The implication in these accounts was that doctors and other staff caused complainants distress by their violation of fundamental and shared normative expectations rather than technical ones.

Complaint letters also anticipate that the complaint may be dismissed as arising from the complainant's ignorance, unreasonableness or complaining nature rather than more objectively from the event or circumstances. Lloyd-Bostock and Mulcahy (1994) found that statements pre-empting that conclusion included assertions that: 'I don't usually complain' (16 letters); 'I don't like to complain' (14 letters); 'I felt I had to write' (25 letters); mentioning that others also felt that something worthy of complaint had happened (50 letters); or praising other visits or other aspects of the hospital stay (76 letters). Statements anticipating justifications can also be understood as pre-empting dismissal of the complaint by displaying that the complainant has considered the hospital's point of view and still regarded the matter as complaint-worthy. Mention of attempts to put matters right were common and implied that the complainant did not complain lightly and had tried to remedy matters before resorting to complaining. Less frequent categories found by Lloyd-Bostock and Mulcahy (1994) included statements about the complainant's status (32 letters), medical knowledge or contacts. In addition, many (25 per cent) mentioned difficulties and problems that were not part of the substance of the complaint, such as the continued ill health of the patient, or difficulties coping at home. Lloyd-Bostock (1999) argues that while apparently irrelevant to the complaint, these statements suggested an obligation on the part of the hospital to reply sympathetically. Allsop's (1994) analysis of letters of complaint also places emphasis on the ways in which complaints from relatives seek to protect their good name as competent lay health workers. Her work draws attention to the importance of moral identities among those who care for the ill and the way in which a failure in a treatment programme prompts them to justify their own part in caring for the patient. As the majority of complaints made on behalf of a patient are made by women, her analysis also has a significance for our understanding of the role of gender and kinship in these accounts.[16]

What do complainants seek to achieve?

Understanding what complainants want to achieve is also important if grievance resolution systems are to be effective and the financial threat posed by complaints accurately assessed. Complaints and claims are commonly discussed outside consumer networks as attempts to obtain a material remedy of some kind. Lawyers in particular tend to view them as a call for compensation. In part this is explained by the fact that the civil justice system converts all injury into a financial sum and does not explicitly offer more creative remedies for litigants. The majority of lawyers interviewed for Mulcahy et al.'s (1999) study of mediation even argued that the obtaining of non-financial or 'soft' remedies was not part of their job. Complaints systems have traditionally been considerably more flexible in the remedies they can offer but it is not uncommon for complainants to be characterized as being on a 'fishing expedition' for evidence which would allow them to make a claim for compensation. However, a number of research studies across the different settings of family practice and hospitals, using different methodologies, have shown that most people place an emphasis on non-financial remedies. In addition, it is clear that many complaints cannot even be labelled instrumental in the sense of requesting a particular outcome.

Despite the popular image within medical circles of complainants and litigants being revenge and compensation hungry, Allsop's (1994) study of ten years' worth of primary care (127) complaints to one medical service committee found only a minority of complainants wanted to prevent the doctor from practising (2 per cent); punish the doctor (9 per cent); and that only 6 per cent mentioned suing or the possibility of suing. The main aims expressed in their letters were to get an explanation and investigation (29 per cent); stop a poor standard of practice (22 per cent); or simply voice their grievance (20 per cent). More recently Kyffin et al.'s (1997) study of the complaints made to 12 hospital Trusts confirms that non-material goals continue to motivate patients and their relatives to complain and that retribution is but a low priority. In their study, as many as 74 per cent of respondents claimed that they complained in order to prevent a reoccurrence. Others wanted to obtain an explanation (49 per cent) or an apology (28 per cent). By way of contrast, only 4 per cent were interested in instigating disciplinary action. Two-thirds (66 per cent) stressed that they merely wanted to make their dissatisfaction known.

Lloyd-Bostock and Mulcahy's (1994) analysis of 342 letters of complaint to acute hospitals also sought to clarify the extent to which complaints are instrumental in the sense of aiming to achieve some clear further goal beyond the expression of dissatisfaction. Their emphasis was not only on what complainants wanted to achieve but the extent to which a direct request for a particular remedy even formed a part of their protest. In their analysis any statement of what the complainant wanted the hospital to do, however vague or general, was coded and classified. Four main categories emerged from this research. These were specific requests that something should be done to put matters right for this complainant or patient (16 per cent);[17] requests that steps should be taken to put matters right for others in the future (20 per cent);[18] requests relating to the provision of information about what had gone wrong, including asking the hospital to conduct an investigation (21 per cent); and, in just over one-fifth of letters, only 'vague' requests that the hospital should 'resolve the matter', or 'take some action'. Sixty-three letters (21 per cent) contained statements of this kind, and in 67 of these there was no other codeable statement of what the complainant wanted. Thus, in 165 letters (48 per cent) there was either no statement at all or only a vague reference to what the complainant wanted to achieve. These findings seriously challenge the image of the overly-adversarial, compensation-seeking complainant but support the argument made in the previous chapter that voiced complaints are often still immature grievances. They also suggest that the opportunity to call doctors to account and the protection of dignity and moral identity can be more important than material gain.

The emphasis on material goals is also obvious when it comes to considering the needs and motivation of claimants. Where litigation is concerned there is a particular emphasis on obtaining a financial award as this is the key way the civil justice system has found to remedy the harm caused by negligent activity. As a result, claimants are forced to make a claim for compensation when formally lodging their grievance as a statement of claim. However, the claimant in a medical negligence action may, ironically, not particularly wish for compensation and may be frustrated by out of court settlement of a case if it ends without them having achieved their other goals (Lloyd-Bostock 1999). In their study of medical negligence claimants, Genn and Lloyd-Bostock (1995) found that although compensation ranked comparatively highly in what claimants said they wanted, a quest for compensation was far from being the sole motivation.[19] Seventy-three per cent of the 106 claimants surveyed named something other than compensation or meeting financial needs as their most important purpose in making the claim. Moreover, when discussing financial compensation, claimants often did so in the context of meeting a particular need or making good a significant financial loss caused by the medical mishap such as recompense for business losses or nursing care. As with complaints it was much less common for claimants to justify making a claim in terms of the need for redress or retribution (Genn and Lloyd-Bostock 1995; Lloyd-Bostock 1999). Similarly in Vincent et al.'s (1994) study of the reasons why people sue their doctors it was found that between 40 and 49 per cent of claimants surveyed wanted an apology or to make health providers understand what had happened and that 50 per cent wanted an admission of fault. When asked what would have prevented them from taking legal action, the same respondents cited an explanation or apology; the correction of the mistake; the payment of compensation; or the admission of negligence. In response to such findings, the National Audit Office (2001) has expressed concern that those hand-ling clinical negligence claims are too narrowly focused on certain types of remedies during the settlement process. They have concluded that solicitors and claims managers are also not accustomed to offering creative packages and that this was likely to lead to frustrated claims and dissatisfaction.

These findings are also reflected in Mulcahy et al.'s (1999) study of the needs of medical negligence claimants which draws on the findings of the earlier work reported here. This survey of 117 claimants found that at the outset of their case claimants had an extensive range of goals other than a quest for damages. The categories of remedies they cited included steps to stop the same thing happening to someone else (52 per cent); the provision of an apology (44 per cent); an opportunity to make the other side understand their concerns (40 per cent); for someone to show that they cared (35 per cent); an opportunity to hear what the other side had to say (28 per cent); to talk through all the issues (27 per cent); arrangements to be made for treatment (27 per cent); and an opportunity to meet the other side face to face (25 per cent). When asked to prioritize their aims, an even smaller proportion than in Genn and Lloyd-Bostock's (1995) study cited compensation as their first priority (36 per cent) and this was followed most closely by a desire to prevent recurrence of the medical mishap (27 per cent). In the words of one of the claimants who took part in the survey:

> The money can't completely resolve it. The money doesn't make up for the person you love. Money can't give you an explanation. That's what you need. It settles your brain cells and you can get on with your life thinking, 'Yeah, they told me this and they told me that'. My solicitor didn't understand the need to be told. Money won't keep me from worrying and thinking . . . thinking, thinking, thinking, will it?
> (Mulcahy 2000: 42)

What emerges from these studies is not only that complainants and claimants want a wider range of remedies than the systems they use are equipped, disposed or trained to provide, but that process and appropriate responses to voiced grievances are crucial to our understanding of how to make these systems more responsive.

Addressing the concerns of patients and their relatives

Elsewhere it has been suggested that whatever the quality of technical care it is most often a failure to treat a person as deserving of attention, time or dignity which acts as a catalyst in the decision to voice a grievance (Allsop and

Mulcahy 1996). If this is the case, it seems likely that the grievance will not be fully addressed if attention, time or respect do not form part of the response or processing of the grievance. The DoH's official evaluation of the complaints procedure introduced in 1996 shows, for instance, that the poor attitudes of staff, a lack of respect and inadequate explanations made a considerable contribution to the fact that two-thirds of complainants they contacted were dissatisfied with the handling of complaints and three-quarters found the process stressful and distressing (Posnett et al. 2001). Dissatisfaction with responses to complaints is clearly not uncommon.[20]

It has been argued above that patients want a wide range of remedies and that in some cases they want nothing more than to make a protest. Whatever their motivation, all complainants appear to crave good processing of their dispute. Process has considerable potential to render the complainant more dignified or to further exacerbate the original indignity complained about. Posnett et al. (2001) found that a major source of dissatisfaction among complainants was that the process was neither fair nor impartial but was felt to be biased in favour of staff. In evaluating the same system, the PLP anticipated the importance of process and used the principles of natural justice as its gold standard in evaluating the current procedure. A key concern of the researchers was the fact that, while Trusts have a separate department for dealing with complaints, complainants with a grievance against a GP were commonly expected to complain directly to the person they thought responsible for inadequate care. Complainants in the study were fearful of retribution such as being struck off a GP's list and felt daunted by having to confront the person concerned. Many were understandably extremely sceptical about whether they would receive an honest or impartial answer (Wallace and Mulcahy 1999). Participants in the PLP research also felt strongly that there were insufficient mechanisms in place to deal appropriately with complaints that raise serious questions about performance, conduct or competence that places patients at risk. It was in these cases that the credibility of local resolution was most undermined and its appropriateness questioned. Participants' level of dissatisfaction with the process indicated a pressing need for alternative procedures to local resolution which would allow for early referral to more independent investigatory and remedial processes.

In their study of 12 hospital Trusts in the north-west, Kyffin et al. (1997) found that over 75 per cent of complainants said that they were dissatisfied with the response of the Trust. In particular, formal response letters failed to address all their concerns. Complainants were not alone in these negative evaluations. CHCs also thought that procedures were daunting for complainants and that the flexibility of the procedures brought unpredictability. This was particularly so within the family practitioner sector where the formal requirements for processing complaints are minimal (DoH 2001). Similarly, in the PLP study, complainants spoke of the struggle involved in obtaining a satisfactory response to their complaint, concerns about not being believed and also of the frustration at the length of time it took to deal with their complaint. Lloyd-Bostock and Mulcahy (1994) found that, even when an apology was given, the elements of a full apology were often not present with the result that the hospital's response appeared insincere. Moreover, 36 per cent of the 98 complainants interviewed rated the hospital as 'not at all' accepting responsibility for the event complained of and 57 per cent rated the hospital as 'very much' or 'rather' trying to defend itself. Forty-one per cent said that they had been given an unsatisfactory explanation.[21]

The results indicate the importance of an appropriate social response to the complaint. It is evidently important to complainants that their complaint be acknowledged and taken seriously, and that the hospital accepts responsibility. Lloyd-Bostock and Mulcahy (1994) found a particularly strong positive correlation between satisfaction and the patient's belief that the hospital intended to improve things for the future. This finding suggests that when complainants state that they are complaining in order to prevent others suffering in the future, they genuinely wish for this and are not merely justifying their complaint with reference to altruistic goals. It also confirms that if an apology is to fulfil a mitigating and conciliatory function then doctors or hospitals need to give substance to explanations and statements of remorse by conceding that matters are unsatisfactory and indicating, credibly, that they intend to take remedial action.

In a later article on the subject, Lloyd-Bostock (1999) argued that the same model could in principle apply as much to legal claims as it could to complaints. Although a number of different considerations apply to claims, complainants and claimants frequently express similar purposes or goals, and a view of claims as a quest for compensation is too narrow. By comparing data from her complaints study with Mulcahy (Mulcahy and Lloyd-Bostock 1994) with her later study of claims conducted with Genn (Genn and Lloyd-Bostock 1995), Lloyd-Bostock argues that a similar pattern emerges and that claimants, like complainants, frequently express dissatisfaction with the response of the hospital or doctor. They report encountering defensiveness, not being taken seriously and being treated in a dismissive or patronizing manner. Eighty-three per cent of respondents in the later study of claims said they had 'a lot of difficulty' obtaining information and another 11 per cent said they had encountered 'some difficulty'. Asked whether the doctor was defensive, 74 per cent reported 'very much' and 80 per cent rated as 'definitely true' the statement that the medical profession was protecting itself. When asked whether the doctor took their concerns seriously, 51 per cent chose the most extreme response of 'not at all' (Lloyd-Bostock 1999).

Mulcahy et al. (1999) have suggested that the dissatisfaction associated with poor handling of a claim is far from temporary. Their findings, which are summarized in Figure 5.1, have demonstrated that when claimants' goals

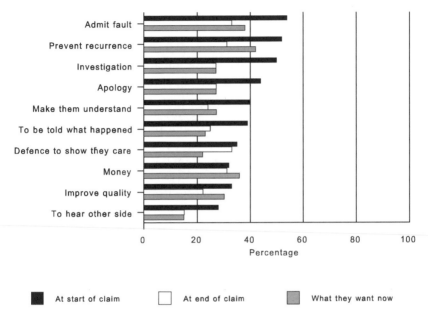

Figure 5.1 What plaintiffs wanted over time

Source: Mulcahy et al. 1999.

are charted over time, and claimants are given the opportunity to reflect on the handling of their claim between 2 and 7 years after first registering it, many claimants' needs remained unmet. Indeed, by the end of their claim, their needs for a range of remedies actually *increased*. This suggests that while the aims of a portion of claimants are satisfied, there is incomplete closure of many grievances despite the fact that plaintiffs may have exhausted formal grievance procedures.

Conclusion

When complainants voice their grievances about doctors, they run the risk of becoming 'bad' or 'problem' patients or carers because they violate the norms of the medical relationship which expect them not to make trouble or interrupt established medical routines. In doing so they no longer fulfil their 'role' as passive and dependent. The challenge posed by this form of protest gives complainants a central role in which they are empowered to initiate a process of investigation which can be time-consuming and stressful for the doctor complained about. Complainants also retain the discretion to abandon the complaint should they wish to do so, a privilege not afforded doctors within the grievance structures reviewed here. In modern societies, these forms of activism and calling to account are increasingly accepted as legitimate and have even come to be encouraged by policy makers. A number of high profile investigations of medical error and abuse initiated by complainants have reinforced the contention that they can contribute to the regulation of medical work.

It is clear that complainants experience strong emotional reactions to the circumstances leading to complaints and the processing of them. Caplan (1995) points to the limited work which has been undertaken in this field as evidence that recognition of the high emotion involved in disputes renders it unlikely that resolution will be achieved. This is a view which is not palatable to those who believe that the natural and proper end to dispute resolution should be peace and settlement. Elsewhere much anthropological work on disputes has been criticized because of the expectation that third-party intervention should lead to harmony. But it would appear that disputes are often not resolved to the satisfaction of both parties and that this will also have an impact on the possibility of 'emotional closure'. I have attempted to show in this chapter that complainants are often left with a residue of dissatisfaction long after the complaint is considered closed by the organization handling it. Viewed in this way it may be that grievances and disputes are never completely relegated to the past because they constantly remain unsettled or affect future thresholds of tolerance.

Moreover, while there are empowering aspects of complaining, complainants are often made vulnerable when they voice their grievance. They are defensive about their right to complain and their part in the circumstances which led to their dissatisfaction. They pre-empt the criticisms likely to be made of them and in some cases are so sensitive to claims that they may lack the authority to call doctors to account that they focus their formal complaint on administrative or 'hotel' services over which they can claim more knowledge. I have argued that complainants and claimants are less demanding than is often assumed. Many of their goals do not relate to compensation and a remarkable number of complaints are not instrumental. Despite this, many complainants anticipate that it is not necessarily what is requested of doctors which represents the major challenge but that they have the audacity to complain at all. The accounts of complainants described in this chapter represent just one piece of a jigsaw that also involves doctors, managers, administrators and social networks. But it already becomes clear that the stories of individual complainants follow patterns which reflect and sustain cultural, structural and institutional factors which shape the doctor-patient relationship. The very fact that they feel a need to justify a rupture in the normal pattern of interaction attests to this fact. The issue is not that the patient has no power but that the medical role has institutional authority which dominates complaints in the same way it dominates other forms of patient-doctor interaction.

Notes

1 The Patients Forum website lists 62 groups which are members of its network. In a health context, many of these groups have been set up as a result of discontent with single issues such as the management of chronic morbidity or childbirth. The emergence of a more general consumer movement, especially the women's movement, has also provided an impetus for alterations in the ideal form of the doctor-patient relationship such as those called for by the National Childbirth Trust.

2 It has been argued that a better-educated population which did not experience health care provision prior to the setting up of the welfare state has also come to have higher expectations of state provision.

3 Because their cooperation is considered increasingly important during the implementation of policy, consumer groups often rely on exerting pressure through Parliament and the mass media.

4 According to Foucault (1973), medics replaced priests as guardians of constructed social 'realities'.

5 See, for example, Citizen's Charter Unit (1991); Cabinet Office Complaints Task Force (1993a, 1993b, 1994a, 1994b, 1994c, 1994d, 1994e, 1995a, 1995b, 1995c, 1995d); and Harper Mills and von Bolschwing (1995).

6 The classification of complaints as clinical or non-clinical was, of course, extremely important in determining the extent to which the medical profession maintained control over the complaints procedure before 1996. Even this level of 'detail' has not been made available about complaints in the primary care sector.

7 For some, any concern about a clinician fitted the clinical category whereas others were more disposed to classify only those allegations which related to clinical treatment in this way.

8 When studies of the pre-1996 procedures in the two sectors are compared it is clear that allegations in hospital complaints were more likely to focus on communication problems (23 per cent of all allegations), medical care (30 per cent) and hotel services (23 per cent) (Lloyd-Bostock and Mulcahy 1994), while primary care complaints were more likely to focus on failure to visit (30 per cent), failure in diagnosis (26 per cent) or failure to refer to a hospital (18 per cent) (Allsop 1994; see also Owen 1991).

9 This project concentrated on clinical complaints. Consultants in this study were asked to give an indication of the type of allegations made in the clinical complaints they had received. Since there may have been more than one allegation per complaint, or more than one complaint per consultant, it was not anticipated that the number of allegations made would equal the number of complaints or the number of consultants. In fact, respondents did not give details of all allegations and there were more complaints (929) than allegations

specified (767). Where data on complaints and allegations were present, complaints contained an average of 1.9 allegations. Allegation code categories were pre-coded using a coding framework developed in the Harvard Medical Malpractice Study (Brennan et al. 1991) and further developed in a study of complaints by Mulcahy and Lloyd-Bostock (1994). A number of examples of what might fall into each of these categories were given on the questionnaire. Consultants could make their own decisions about which of the eight categories provided best described the allegations against them. They were also given the opportunity to specify complaints that were not covered by these definitions and these were analysed and coded separately – resulting in some of the original categories being expanded.

10   While the study of complainants involved a one-year cohort, consultants in the same area were asked to reflect on complaints received within the past five years.

11   In line with this argument there was a recognition among some respondents in Mulcahy's (2000) study that their perception of allegations would differ from the complainant's account. As one consultant suggested: 'The nature of the complaint usually differs from the complainee's perspective, which in turn changes with time and experience'.

12   Moore asserts that discussions of emotion in disputes tend to present emotional displays as strategic tools. Commentators have rarely allowed for the possibility of uncontrolled emotional explosions. She concludes: 'Of course, strategic action is often involved. But when the stakes are high for the participants, strong feelings may also play their part, not just cool strategies' (1995: 17). In support of such an argument, Felstiner et al. have asserted: 'We believe that the study of dispute processing has been too removed from the actual difficulties and choices that accompany the recognition that one's life is trouble and that relief from trouble is uncertain, contingent and costly' (1980–1: 653).

13   These findings go some way to understanding the logic of those dissatisfied patients who choose not to pursue their grievance because of the additional trauma involved.

14   The most common format for traditional settlement negotiations is that they take place between solicitors through an exchange of letters. Claimants' evaluation of traditional methods shows that they were denied meaningful participation in this model.

15   However, Mulcahy et al. (1999) also observed that solicitors did not think that it was their job to be creative about remedies. Despite these arguments, the National Audit Office (2001) found in its recent study that 80 per cent of Trusts rarely or never offered meetings with clinicians or remedial health care either within or outside the Trust and that perceptions of participants in current systems created barriers to seeking creative solutions.

16   Eighty-two per cent of complaints in her study were made on behalf of others and of these 75 per cent were made by family members, most often a daughter.

17 This included requests that someone should be disciplined, or an apology should be made, or a meeting arranged, as well as requests for appointments, operations and transport arrangements. Fifty-three letters (16 per cent) included at least one statement in this category.

18 Some were quite general but in other cases a specific change to procedures and practices might be suggested for the benefit of others in the future. Also included in this group were statements expressing the hope that the hospital would make use of the information that a complainant had supplied without specifying a particular course of action.

19 Claimants were asked, 'Please give your most important purpose or purposes in making a claim' and were prompted for the 'most important', 'second most important' and 'third most important'.

20 Studies of satisfaction with the litigation system also reveal a considerable amount of dissatisfaction with current procedures. Critics have drawn attention to the impersonality, insensitivity and remoteness of the law, which is perceived as rigid and formal and as forcing the parties into defensive positions. As a result, the system is ill-equipped to deliver an explanation and investigation of what has occurred. The present system for obtaining compensation encourages confrontation and concealment. It has been argued that much of the cost and delay in Anglo-American systems is attributable to the competitiveness and rancour with which modern litigation is conducted (Menkel-Meadow 1996).

21 Complainants interviewed were asked to rate their overall satisfaction with the handling of their complaint on a 10-point scale. It was explained that a score of 5 or less indicated that they were more dissatisfied than satisfied. The average overall rating was 4.8, with 58 per cent of respondents giving a rating of 5 or less. Twenty per cent rated their dissatisfaction at the extreme end of the scale.

6   From fear to fraternity?
Doctors' reactions to being called to account

Introduction

This chapter explores the impact of complaints on doctors and how they come to understand the criticisms made of them. It considers how doctors describe their emotional reactions to complaints and the way in which complaints prompt them to alter their attitudes to providing medical care. An understanding of such reactions is important if the challenge posed by complaints is to be placed in context. The data presented go some way to explaining why some doctors are so passionate about wanting to retain jurisdiction over complaint handling. The previous chapter stressed the huge emotional costs experienced by complainants when they voice a grievance. Here it is argued that the impact on doctors is also significant and long-lasting. For many, the challenge of complaints prompts an identity crisis which causes them to question their competence. This chapter outlines this process together with the ways in which a doctor's sense of identity as a competent expert comes to be reconstructed in the aftermath of the dispute by reference to medical networks.

It is argued that after an initial period of turmoil, doctors come to rationalize the complaining act and externalize blame for the events and circumstances complained about. The process of coming to terms with challenges from patients ultimately relies on recourse to the medical fraternity. Doctors give meaning to the act of complaining by positioning it within a particular illness episode. This allows them to understand complaints by reference to a bio-medical model of care. Commonly, the reconstruction of a positive sense of identity relies on a deconstruction and undermining of both the complainant and complaint. In seeking to rebuild *their* damaged sense of identity, doctors strive to emphasize the differences between their perception of the cause of events and that put forward by the complainant. The data demonstrate that while doctors present themselves as rational scientists they see complainants as putting forward irrational or illogical accounts while they defended their own work in medical terms, and pay little heed to the contrasting discourses and concerns expressed by complainants.

This chapter relies heavily on largely unpublished data from a study of hospital consultants' reactions to complaints which was undertaken by the author. It is in three main parts. The first section discusses doctors' emotional reaction to complaints. This is followed by a discussion of how they come, on reflection, to rationalize and make sense of complaints. In the final section there is a discussion of how they use networks of professional support in their attempts to find ways of coping with complaints.

Reactions to complaints

The making of a complaint or claim clearly has the potential to prompt strong reactions among doctors because it challenges the core assumption that health care professionals heal or alleviate pain. Basic tenets of the relationships between patients and doctors, and managers and doctors, are called into question and this can lead to a breach of trust, suspicion and anger (Mulcahy and Rosenthal 1999). Although little work on doctors' reactions to complaints has been undertaken in a medical context, research on reactions to other criticisms of medical work suggests ways in which responses are framed and understood. Studies of reactions to mistakes and mishaps demonstrate that intense responses to these events have to be understood within the context of the 'perfectibility model' to which doctors are taught to aspire in the course of their education (Nathanson 1999). Doctors are trained to function at high levels of proficiency and are socialized in medical schools to strive for error-free practice. On the one hand this can lead to psychological defences against admitting errors and on the other to an anxiety about dealing with allegations of poor practice.

Commentators have suggested that doctors are often emotionally devastated by medical mishaps, complaints and medical negligence claims (Allsop 1994; Mulcahy et al. 1996a; Allsop and Mulcahy 1998; Jain and Ogden 1999). Research has demonstrated that doctors are likely to experience a host of symptoms characteristic of stress-induced illness in response to legal claims (Charles 1984). Lavery (1988) has drawn an analogy between these reactions and grief reactions following the death of a close family member. It is clear that many doctors take litigation as a personal affront and argue that this can cause a loss of enjoyment of their professional work (Charles 1984; Charles and Kennedy 1988). Doctors have reported insomnia, appetite change, irritability, headaches and many other symptoms of stress as responses to having made mistakes (Ennis and Grudzinskas 1993). Despite the intensity of reactions, they have demonstrated a reluctance to get help from psychiatrists or counsellors, most commonly because it could be viewed as a sign of weakness

(Ennis and Grudzinskas 1993; Nathanson 1999). In their review of the literature on doctors' responses to medical mishap and negligence, Ennis and
Vincent (1994) have suggested that feelings of anger and betrayal are not
unusual in doctors reporting on the personal effects of litigation. They place
particular emphasis on the feelings of isolation caused by claims and the ways
in which litigation and the threat of a lawsuit subtly change doctors' relationships with all patients and not just those who actually initiate claims against
them.

Do doctors react in the same way to complaints? Mulcahy's (2000) study,
based on a questionnaire to 848 hospital consultants in the Oxford region
found that complaints have a significant and often long-term impact on
doctors. The ten most frequently mentioned responses to a complaint were all
negative. These were irritation (52 per cent); worry (42 per cent); concern (38
per cent); surprise (38 per cent); annoyance (37 per cent); anger (33 per cent);
distress (32 per cent); disappointment (31 per cent); anxiety (28 per cent); and
vulnerability (28 per cent).[1] In their written accounts of emotional reactions,
consultants in the study spoke of complaints as unwelcome intrusions and
improper demands. Complaint handling was not seen as an integral part of
what they did but the cause of extra work which got in the way of more
important technical tasks. Consultants in this group were far from recognizing
a prima facie right of complainants to hold them to account. Rather, they
characterized complaining as a morally reprehensible activity which had an
adverse effect on their ability to care for other, more worthy patients.

Interviews indicated that consultants found complaints upsetting and
hurtful because they implied that a patient had questioned their competence
and commitment, and this in turn had affected their perception of themselves
as competent professionals.[2] More specifically, Mulcahy (2000) suggests that
consultants go through a number of different stages in coming to terms with
complaints. The stages are eloquently outlined in a quotation from one of the
consultants she interviewed. In his words:

> When doctors receive complaints they go through a series of emo-
> tions. First of all they are frightened, because it is the beginning of a
> process they don't understand. Then they feel injured, because they
> feel they are only doing their best or the complainant does not under-
> stand what they have done. Where the complaint is unjustified they
> feel irritation. Finally, they get round to asking the most important
> question: Is this complaint actually about the standard of clinical
> care?

An initial feeling of fear or isolation was a common response among
the sample. Somewhat surprisingly given their high social status and situational power, many doctors also experienced a feeling of loss of control or

powerlessness, of complainants being 'unsatisfiable', of being under siege. In part this was accounted for by the fact that it is within the power of complainants to both initiate and pursue complaints. GPs reflect what Scott and Lyman (1968: 52) have called 'sad tales'. In the words of one of Mulcahy's (2000) respondents: 'The greatest sense is of futility – why bother to try when resources are inadequate and patients are complaining?'

Emotional responses varied according to the facts of the case, whether the complaint was considered justified, or with the passing of time. It was particularly noticeable that the impact of complaints on consultants was much greater and longer-lasting where doctors felt that the grievances of patients were wholly or partly unjustified. Interestingly, the emotions they described reflected the type of haunting described by complainants in the previous chapter. One consultant explained: 'The complaints that have the greatest impact are those which are unjustified. If a complaint is justified, then there is a clear route for you to take. You apologize and improve your practice. Where it is unjustified, you are left to mull it over, and over, and over, and over . . .' Consultants in this 'unjustified' category were five times as likely to feel disappointment or anxiety; four times as likely to feel vulnerability, irritation, annoyance or anger; and three times as likely to be worried, concerned, distressed or surprised.

Despite their feelings of vulnerability, many doctors in Mulcahy's study made strong counter allegations against complaints, and described *their* desire for redress. A number drew attention to the fact that while complainants could expect redress if their complaint was justified, the same opportunity was not afforded to consultants when complaints were considered unjustified. In the words of one consultant:

> The problem is that there is no real mechanism for redress. We say we know that some complaints aren't justified, but we can never really make our views known. There should be a mechanism to deal with frivolous complaints. Doctors want their say as well. If someone is wrong, then that has to be said publicly as well. I thought of going to a solicitor to sue the complainant for defamation. But that would have caused weeks of misery. I wanted to get my own back.

And another explained: 'It's not that I want to fine them or anything, but the relationship is so one-sided. They have done the damage as soon as they make the complaint. All we can do is sue for defamation.' And again: 'The hospital complaints system does not reject complaints. It absorbs them. We are never defended. Our actions are explained, but they are not defended.' These quotations highlight a tension which exists when designing any internal complaints system. Should the complaints system be seen as part of a service to patients and relatives which addresses their concerns in a way which satisfies them, or should it be a 'wrong-righting' activity which judges the respective merits of opposing versions of events? Interview data suggest that, while doctors could accept that satisfying the complainant may be an expedient way to deal with the complaints and reduce the risk of escalation, denial of adjudication is considered unjust and appeared to rankle long after the complaint has been dealt with.

The perception of the broader threat posed by individual complaints is also important to consider. The strength of doctors' reactions partly relates to a loss of control over a process that might eventually expose them to disciplinary systems such as that operated by the GMC and the courts. It is not just the incidence of complaints which threatens doctors but their capacity to render criticism more visible. If disputes are pursued beyond the first stage of the complaints procedure, they are likely to be drawn to the attention of senior medical colleagues and may well affect a doctor's career prospects. Although relatively rarely used, the threat of formal sanctions and loss of reputation throws a shadow over those who receive complaints. The potential for complaints to evolve into legal claims has been shown to overshadow complaint handling and fuels the construction of complaints as a more significant problem than might at first be assumed. Mulcahy (2000) found that fear of litigation posed a significant threat to doctors who had only been complained about and that consultants treated complaints and claims as synonymous. As one explained: 'Of course, we worry. We worry all the time. And it is there every time you formulate your response to complainants. Whilst wanting to deal sensitively with a sensitive topic, you have to make sure you are not admitting anything or encouraging them to pursue'. When doctors in this study (Mulcahy 2000) and a study of GPs (Allsop and Mulcahy 1998) were asked what they thought complainants wanted, most recognized that explanations, apologies and investigations were important. But many more GPs perceived complainants to want a reprimand and more hospital consultants said complainants wanted compensation than was reported in studies of complainants' desires (see, in particular, Lloyd-Bostock and Mulcahy 1994; Lloyd-Bostock 1999).

Fears overshadowing the handling of complaints and claims also went beyond the potential for exposure to wider concerns about broader cultural and attitudinal shifts in society. Law and the discourse of rights has also come to be seen as a constraint on clinical autonomy rather than facilitative of it (Dingwall 1994). In Mulcahy's (2000) study, images of an impending crisis were not uncommon. In part, this was blamed on a policy environment which encourages criticism of doctors but the majority of consultants surveyed and interviewed also expressed concerns that the *Citizen's Charter* initiative had encouraged patients to complain. As one consultant neurologist argued: 'We are just under more and more pressure from patients and what really gets to me is that patients are being told to complain. It's all got out of proportion.

The number of complaints has rocketed as has the amount of time we spend on them ... everybody is using up their time on them.' Brown and Simanowitz suggest that the 'mere hint of negligence may lead to a knee jerk reaction of determined defence' (1995: 488).[3] Similarly, in an American context McQuade (1991) comments that the perceived threat of litigation has almost as much impact on clinical practice as an actual lawsuit.

In the UK, Summerton (1995) found in his survey of GPs that doctors made significant changes to their practice to avert complaints. Common practices were an increase in diagnostic testing, an increased referral rate and follow-up, more detailed patient explanations and more detailed note-taking. Some of these practices could lead to benefits for patients, leading Summerton to use the terms 'positive' and 'negative defensive medicine' to describe them.[4] Mulcahy et al. (1996a) and Jain and Ogden (1999) all found that doctors changed their practice to avert complaints in a positive way. In a former study, doctors reported changes were made to increase the amount of information in record keeping, liaison with other agencies and staff training; and to review out-of-hours cover and appointment systems.[5] Mulcahy's study of hospital consultants found, in common with Summerton's (1995) research, that better record/note-keeping and fuller consultations with patients featured quite prominently among the reactions described by the sample group. One hundred and fifty-seven (64 per cent) consultants specified 371 ways in which their medical practice had changed.[6] While some of responses which emerged, such as avoidance of certain patients and increased wariness, may be suggestive of a more negative approach to the provision of treatment, the data tend to support the proposition that long-term reactions to complaints may be inappropriately characterized as 'defensive'. Significantly, Mulcahy also found a strong correlation between the intensity of emotional response and the propensity to change practice – doctors with stronger emotional reactions to complaints were more likely to alter their clinical practice. Interestingly, those who made no change in practice recorded fewer emotional responses to the complaint than those who did. This suggests that in contrast to the crisis scenario suggested above, a strong emotional reaction to complaints is far from a problem in the long term and may actually yield the most positive effects.

How do doctors make sense of complaints?

There are a host of theoretical frameworks which might be used to analyse how doctors make sense of complaints. As with complainants, sociological studies suggest that doctors' defences to complaints could be interpreted as part of the social process of impression management (Goffman 1961, 1967), as accounts which provide justifications and excuses (Scott and Lyman 1968) or in the context of the politics of identity (Giddens 1991). Social psychologists have also applied attribution theory to explain how disputants come to terms with criticism and construct defences (Lloyd-Bostock and Mulcahy 1994). At its simplest, the theory suggests that people prefer to find meaning and order in the world and usually develop explanations of why events happen and why people behave as they do. Despite the variety of theoretical approaches it has been argued that there are a number of common responses when people seek to attribute cause for untoward events, which are related to awarding responsibility and blame to themselves, others or to fate (Tedeschi and Reiss 1981).[7] According to Weiner et al.'s (1972) three-dimensional model, for instance, there are a number of ways of classifying responsibility for any given phenomena. Perceived causes of outcome can vary in terms of being: external (something about the environment) or internal (something about the individual); stable (not capable of changing in the future) or unstable (capable of change); intentional (foreseen, wilful) or unintentional (not consciously desired). Empirical studies of complaints and medical mishaps demonstrate quite visibly that, in a medical context, the preference is for explanations of cause which place emphasis on external factors. This is demonstrated by using the data collected and reported by Allsop (1994), Ennis and Vincent (1994) and Lloyd-Bostock and Mulcahy (1994) to fill in the fields suggested by Weiner et al. (1972) (see Figure 6.1).

It is clear from Figure 6.1 that doctors who have participated in these projects have rarely internalized blame for mishaps or grievances. Where they accept some responsibility, they tend to view fault as unintentional. Problems with framing responses to criticisms in these ways have been identified by Tennen and Affleck (1990) who suggest, in their wide-ranging review of the social-psychological literature on this topic that blaming others for threatening events is dysfunctional and suggests impaired psychological well-being. Similarly, Ennis and Grudzinskas (1993) have suggested that unwarranted generalizations about patients as a whole can result in perceptual distortions in the doctor-patient relationship.

Researchers have found that doctors use a number of different devices to externalize blame for events or circumstances complained about. A common trend is for doctors to infer that it is the complainant's inability to come to terms with what has happened that is the real cause of the grievance. Empirical studies suggest that they are typically described as irrational in contrast to the rational doctor. One of the most popular caricatures of complainants to emerge from empirical studies is the problem patient (see Rosenthal et al. 1980; Richman 1987) – an example of the condemned condemning the condemners (Scott and Lyman 1968). Mulcahy (2000) found that for many consultants the cause of complaint was not seen as bad care but the personality of the complainant. One consultant summed up this stance:

INTENTIONAL		
	Internal	**External**
Stable		Greedy lawyers Lack of funding in service Distortion by media Unreal expectations of medicine Complainants are selfish
Unstable		The complainant had not carried out lay medical work properly

UNINTENTIONAL		
	Internal	**External**
Stable	Ignorance of regulations and responsibilities	The uncertainty of the disease process The uncertainty of medical work Outside of their contractual obligations
Unstable	Pressures of work	Traffic jams or the weather caused delays

Figure 6.1 Examples of attribution in a medical setting applying Weiner et al.'s (1972) three-dimensional model to the work of Allsop (1994), Ennis and Vincent (1994) and Lloyd-Bostock and Mulcahy (1994)

> You could do a psychological profile of patients coming into hospital and select those who were likely to complain before giving them any clinical care. Critical incident analysis is a much better way to identify adverse events. Too many mistakes are *not* complained about. Complaints are nebulous events involving perceived deficiencies of care.

Mulcahy found that positive or empathetic comments about complainants were made in just 6 out of 141 commentaries on why people complained. Complainants were most often described in negative or dismissive terms as 'moaners', 'nasty', 'abusers' and 'malcontents'. Interestingly, 21 consultants, only 12 of whom were specialists in psychiatric medicine, described complainants as exhibiting symptoms of psychiatric illness such as 'personality disorders', 'paranoia' and 'neuroticism'.

Mulcahy's work suggests that doctors also make considerable use of recourse to notions of scientific truth in coming to terms with complaints. She argues that a scientific account of complaints leads the doctor to argue that there are objective signs which explain the dissatisfaction experienced by the complainant while negating the threat posed to the doctor. Allsop (1994) has also stressed the ways in which the defences offered serve to defend the doctor's professional identity by making references to considered clinical judgement, the opinions of other doctors, their normal practice or their qualifications. Allsop concludes that doctors display certainty about their clinical judgement while using the uncertainty of the disease process as a defence.[8] Like complainants, they defended their position by shifting blame and, in doing so, often stepped outside the parameters of professional detachment to attack the identity of complainants. In these situations the complainant's feeling of being aggrieved is presented as a physical manifestation of disease. The presentation of scientific 'facts' of this kind makes it difficult for the logic of their justification to be questioned, and indeed this is the purpose of the construction.

It could be argued that by labelling the complainant as 'sick' the doctor no longer deals with an individual consciously attacking them but a dual personality who is sincerely complaining while unconsciously coming to terms with disease and its treatment. The complainant is transformed into a passive and objectified being who does not *know*. In this way it can be argued that it is the doctor rather than the complainant who is getting at the 'real' problem (Dodier 1994). If the cause of the dissatisfaction can be understood by reference to disease then the validity of the complaint as a challenge to the doctor's world is undermined and this allows the doctor to present him/herself as someone who did not cause the problem but can solve it. This construction is especially interesting given that studies have shown that around 60 per cent of complaints to hospitals are made by someone other than a patient undergoing medical care (Lloyd-Bostock and Mulcahy 1994). In this way both the diseased and the healthy became medicalized.

Data from Mulcahy's (2000) study provide some excellent examples of attempts to attribute a scientific or medical, rather than a fault-based, cause to complaints. Consultants argued that it was the specialty involved in the care, rather than fault, that was the most likely indicator of a propensity to complain.[9] Interviewees drew attention to the fact that each specialty has its own characteristics, working practices, environment, equipment and connections with other services. Each deals with distinctive clinical problems and needs which explain a greater propensity to complain about certain types of care. The likelihood of a particular illness or treatment prompting complaints was linked to five particular factors: whether the diagnosis or treatment involved the imparting of bad news; the length and intensity of the treatment episode; the level of uncertainty involved in care; the serious consequences of mistakes; and the emotional investment involved in particular types of treatment.

Respondents explained that specialties involving terminal care and diagnosis, such as oncology and general medicine, where bad news was regularly imparted, were in particular danger of suffering from the emotional aftermath of communicating a poor prognosis. Conversely, they argued that 'good news' specialties such as orthodontics had fewer complaints.[10] In their use of this term they were describing specialists' capacity and ability to improve or cure. One consultant, specializing in general medicine, remarked:

We are definitely a bad news specialty. Young patients often die unexpectedly and there is a lot of guilt at the death. When it comes to it, people do not know how to deal with it and their obvious reaction is to channel the emotions onto someone else. It's a case of shooting the messenger.[11]

The length of the relationship – or 'at-risk' period – with the patient was also highlighted as important by the study. Paradoxically, doctors argued that the longer the 'at-risk' period the less likely it was that a complaint would be received because with frequent contact the patient was much better able to place episodes of unsatisfactory care within the context of a generally satisfactory service. A good example of this was said to be nephrology where a relationship with a patient could last 20 years. Conversely, accident and emergency specialists were expected to get a lot of complaints because of the abrupt and emotionally charged nature of their interactions with patients. Other specialties were thought to attract complaints because of the risks and uncertainties involved and the difficulties of conveying these notions to patients.

In her study of general practice complaints, Allsop (1994) found that almost one-fifth (18 per cent) of doctors explained untoward events by reference to the claim that uncertainty in medical practice had made outcomes difficult to predict. The problem of uncertainty in medicine has been stressed repeatedly by medical sociologists. Fox (1957) claims that three types of uncertainty disturb physicians: their own incomplete knowledge; the limitations in medical knowledge; and an inability to distinguish between their own ignorance and that of the science they practise. The problem of handling uncertainty in the disease process and how it affects individuals has been seen as a central aspect of learning to be a doctor. However, the 'problem' of uncertainty is handled differently at different stages of a medic's career. While risk and unpredictability may emerge as a key theme in the academic stage of training, practice-based instruction is much more likely to place emphasis on the benefit of confidence about the outcomes of medical interventions when dealing with clients (Allsop 1994). It is interesting to reflect that doctors revert to explanations founded on the uncertainty of medical work in the defence work they undertake in reactions to complaints. Where complaints relate to the process of communicating prognosis and risk it can be imagined how such reactions could also serve to exacerbate the complainant's sense of grievance.

Many doctors in Mulcahy's (2000) study described the dilemmas involved. They argued that although they had been consulted as experts that expertise was then questioned. They described the difficulties they experienced in coming to terms with their expert advice not being accepted. Some doctors reflected on the need to make a fair and balanced judgement of risks. But they were also aware that there were pressures on them from the patients to provide a definite diagnosis in the face of inevitable clinical uncertainty. A number described the ways in which professional judgement facilitated their isolation. One doctor commented: 'Practising medicine is about exercising judgement, that is why we're so opinionated. But we are vulnerable prima donnas, [we] play solo with patients and have to stand alone by decisions.'

Consultants in Mulcahy's study also argued that in certain specialties the consequences of error were more serious than others and that this increased the propensity to complain about certain types of treatment. Anaesthetics, obstetrics and orthopaedics were all cited as specialties where the effect of mistakes can be life-threatening. As one anaesthetist remarked: 'Mistakes in anaesthesia are all or nothing. If you make a mistake it tends to be a really serious one. In medicine as a whole, doctors are pleased with a 60 per cent response rate, but in anaesthetics that one mistake means that your severity average shoots right up.'

Finally, doctors talked about the impact of high emotional investment by patients and others in the care received. They suggested that in certain specialties such as psychiatry and paediatrics relatives were more likely to complain because they were experiencing guilt or frustration. Looking back to the previous chapter's analysis of who makes complaints, it is clear that the notion of agency is an important one in complaining as many complaints are made by relatives or friends. The idea of such complaints being fuelled by the need to perform a caring role well or shoulder social responsibility is clearly in stark contrast to the description of motivation provided by consultants in Mulcahy's study.

The threat to group or professional identity

In the process of coming to terms with complaints, doctors attach considerable importance to a sense of group identity and professional values. Group ideology is seen as performing a legitimating function by protecting the established order as well as being a shield from internal conflict or outside challenges, such as complaints. The concept of a group may be overly simplistic since doctors practise within specialties, sub-specialties, thought collectives, segments and disciplines, all of which may have different ideologies and missions and may be in conflict. Reflecting on the political struggles in setting up the NHS and complaints procedures, it has been argued in earlier chapters that the assumption of homogeneity of views and a joint sense of identity may be misplaced. Some scholars, such as Bucher and Strauss (1960–1), have preferred to describe professions as loose amalgamations of segments, only delicately held together, pursuing different objectives in different manners. Other empirical studies have suggested that despite images of a large and efficient network there is little evidence to show that ideas are circulated and exchanged even between groups of medical specialists (Arksey 1994) although thought-styles may nonetheless unite them. The notion of group is also problematic when it comes to distinguishing group ideas and ideologies from those held by individuals within them (Linnea Schneid 1994), and from those held by wider groups or environments. Despite these reservations, many factors serve to reinforce a collective sense of identity among doctors including their long training, the intense socialization process, the role of patronage in career development, the framework of self-regulation, the web of promotional organizations and activities, the collegiate setting of much work practice and the norm of clinical autonomy. These create the conditions for work shelter, but also the incentives for identity maintenance and for professional politics in a wide range of institutional areas (Allsop and Mulcahy 1998; Rosenthal 1999). In his seminal account of how GPs manage complaints and bad practice, Freidson (1980) argues that physicians have a shared conception of themselves as ethical, conscientious, competent and stable. It is because it was inherent in this set of beliefs about their identity that patients should trust them that doctors in Friedson's study were so severely challenged by complaints.

When reviewing the literature on disputes between doctors and patients it becomes apparent that the challenges of complaints go beyond the particular allegations made to a threat to the symbolic and ceremonial order of doctor-patient interactions. Viewed in this way, criticisms of a doctor's work can often be seen as a criticism of the profession's knowledge base or standards. They can prompt a group (as well as an individual) 'legitimation crisis' because complaints call into question the doctor's technical and moral authority over biomedical knowledge (see Habermas 1976). A complaint may represent a double challenge: to have got something wrong technically and not to have used medical knowledge in the interest of the patient. Moreover, this challenge has come from a lay person who is not considered to be in a position to judge medical work. As Schutz comments: 'the expert . . . knows very well that only a fellow expert will understand all the technicalities and implications of a problem in his field, and he will never accept a lay man or a dilettante as the competent judge of his performance' (1964: 123). Doctors' affinity to the group has been evidenced in two main ways in relation to complaints. First, it is clear that once the initial impact of having received a complaint has been experienced, doctors tend to turn, almost exclusively, to medical networks in their attempts to come to terms with what has happened and understand it. Second, the identity work undertaken when responding to complaints also gives doctors an opportunity to define who is within the group and in doing so reiterate what are considered to be the proper boundaries of professional identity. In the remainder of this section each of these themes is considered in turn.

When individuals are criticized, it is a common reaction to look to others for support and disputants often utilize networks of kin, affinity and close patronage (Caplan 1995). Commentators have identified how support networks can provide emotional backup and act as 'sounding boards'.[12] According to this view, there is a danger in viewing disputes as involving only individuals when important collective interests may be involved which encourage the mobilization of support networks (Felstiner et al. 1980–1; Mulcahy and Tritter 1998). In their review of the anthropological literature, Mather and Yngvesson (1980–81) stress the importance of third parties in providing support and narrowing or expanding the issues involved. They have argued that such transformation of a dispute can involve antagonists and third parties in one or more of three processes. First, that of 'rephrasing' – that is, a reformulation of the issues in dispute into a public discourse. After rephrasing, the new account of the dispute will continue to reflect the perspectives of the antagonists, but it will also reflect the interests of any third parties involved in the rephrasing. Second, 'expansion' involves a challenging of existing established categories for defining the ambit of the dispute. In this way accepted frameworks are 'stretched'. Third, there is 'narrowing', a process through which established categories for classifying events and relationships are imposed in a way which makes it amenable to conventional categories. Narrowing is particularly common among officials in formalized grievance procedures where there are routine-driven ways of handling claims.

Patterns of help-seeking are a form of protection in which individuals may talk to others who share the same framework of meaning and knowledge base. Talking to colleagues and intimate networks of friends and family can act as a rehearsal ground for the account of their behaviour which doctors give to complainants. Help-seeking activity can also act as a form of catharsis which allows them to come to terms with the criticism made. But, in a medical context, writers have emphasized the barriers to doctors approaching others for help. Leape claims that doctors are typically isolated by their emotional responses to medical mishap because there are rarely support networks which can serve to facilitate 'emotional healing for the fallible physician' (1999: 23). Similarly, in their empirical study of house doctors' responses to complaints, Wu et al. (1991) found that only 50 per cent of house officers discussed their most significant mistakes with attending physicians. Other studies have found that doctors often seek informal help and advice by discussing a concern in a lighthearted way in an informal setting but are unlikely to seek help by openly admitting their concerns (Bosk 1982). It has been suggested that the perceived need to be infallible creates a strong pressure towards intellectual dishonesty, to cover up mistakes rather than to admit them (McIntyre and Popper 1989). Nathanson (1999) has argued that a general ethos has traditionally prevailed which discourages doctors from reporting errors or cooperating with investigations of allegations of mistakes by themselves or others. Empirical research has suggested that errors are rarely admitted or discussed because of the fear of censure or that colleagues will regard the subject of the allegations as incompetent. In his study of trainee doctors' ways of rationalizing their mistakes, Mizrahi (1984) found that denial, distancing and discounting were common strategies. In a similar vein, Rosenthal's (1995) work on doctors' reactions to bad practice suggests that a considerable degree of tolerance of deviant activity exists within the medical profession, but that knowledge that colleagues are regularly underperforming can prompt informal regulation of their behaviour by social distancing, extra scrutiny of medical work undertaken, the redirection of work and 'quiet chats'.

However, the suggestion that doctors do not readily seek help when held to account has not been substantiated in a UK setting when complaints and claims, rather than mishaps, are being considered. Mulcahy (2000) found that the majority of consultants in her study (92 per cent) talked to at least one other person about complaints received and only 9 per cent said that they would have liked someone else to talk to. However, the same study did show that doctors are highly selective about who they approach. Professional medical networks were used almost to the exclusion of all others. Other doctors were most often approached for advice (19 per cent); support (17 per cent); information (10 per cent); and in order that feelings could be unburdened (10 per cent) and, significantly, medical colleagues were approached as often as family and friends. One major effect of discussing complaints with colleagues appeared to be that it 'normalizes them'. As one doctor in Mulcahy's study explained:

> When it first happens everything flashes before your eyes. Being disciplined, ridiculed by colleagues, denied promotion and gener- ally thought of as not up to scratch, a bit shoddy. Then you start talking to colleagues and you realise that even if they haven't had a formal complaint patients have made their dissatisfaction felt. I came to see that everyone experiences complaints in one form or another and that most of the time they are ill-founded so why worry?
>
> (2000: 203)

It is interesting to note that consultants were most likely to turn to senior medical colleagues within the same Trust or unit for practical and emotional support of all kinds. This suggests that there is little concern about letting those higher up the medical hierarchy know about the complaint as long as they are doctors working in the same organization. Senior non-medical management, or legal claims advisers, were rarely approached for any type of support or advice (8 per cent). In a similar vein, Mulcahy et al.'s (1996a) small-scale study of 56 GPs' reactions to complaints also found that doctors handling less formal complaints relied heavily on the use of medical support networks, both inside and outside their practice, and rarely went beyond these for advice and emotional support (see also Allsop 1994).[13]

Conclusion

It is clear from the data presented that complaints represent a severe challenge to medical order. They are known to be able to cause a deep and lasting effect on the emotional well-being of those criticized and to affect future relationships with patients. Initially they appear to lead to a disruption or legitimation crisis. Consultants talked about their sense of fear and hurt, of concern about their reputation, of distress at the lack of understanding of their actions and of their vulnerability. The crisis prompted by the challenge to authority most often leads to a recourse to the ideology and support of the other members of medical fraternities. Almost all the consultants in the study had felt it necessary to talk to someone about their concerns and they relied, almost exclusively, on medical colleagues to support their needs. In turn, those complained about strengthened group identity by reiterating what bound those within the group and defining who was outside it. As a result managerial input to responses to complaints was often made impossible and complainants' claims to rationality were questioned.

But the lasting impression is of a discourse employed by medics which was structured to privilege their position. The data presented suggest that the incidence of complaints can be explained in terms of factors associated with disease and the healing process. Complaints were often viewed as part of the emotional aftermath of diagnosis, a stage in patients' coming to terms with their change in status, or prompted by their ignorance of the inevitable risks involved in medical treatment. In this way doctors reverted from being the subjects of criticism to healers with expert diagnostic powers. The model relies on doctors laying claims to a group identity in which medical practice was given an objective reality beyond the actions of individual doctors. In contrast to the unsympathetic images of complainants discussed when consultants were asked to explain their personal reactions to particular complaints about them, the tone of accounts about cause is much more empathetic. This suggests that reference to group ideals provides a more palatable route in attempts to come to terms with criticism. As Cassell (1991) has argued, physicians come to believe that to know the disease and its treatment is to know the illness and treatment of the ill person.

In drawing on the collective identity of the medical group, doctors draw on identities which are familiar and provide some insulation from external challenges to medical work. Both Cohen (1994) and Weeks (1995), in their discussion of group identity, comment on the problem of maintaining common practices and the symbolic re-enactments which reaffirm group identity and difference. Complaints provide an opportunity for group interaction and the demonstration of solidarity as well as providing a sense of belonging through access to networks of support for the individual doctor. The data presented in this chapter suggest that responses to complaints are not isolated events but journeys of response which have an anchor in ever-changing notions of individual, professional and scientific identities.

Many of the emotional responses to complaints outlined above draw attention to the way in which complaints destabilize the expected order in the doctor-patient relationship. Doctors tend to assume that their superior technical knowledge and moral authority is accepted by the health care user but complaints transgress both these norms and, perhaps for this reason, are taken in a personal way as an attack on the self. The accounts of complaints offered by doctors suggest that lay perceptions of unsatisfactory care are given little credence as valid criticism. In an era of consumers, charters and pluralistic approaches to explanations of illness and standards of care, the discourse of patients' rights and the validity of the stories they tell is lacking from explanation about what prompts a challenge to medical care. Instead, the rhetoric of scientific knowledge about illness was used to identify the signs and observable clues of complaints as an offshoot of disease. By seeing complaining as a predictable reaction to disease it becomes a universal phenomenon rather than something that is a personal problem. In claiming the expertise to identify these clues, the consultants in Mulcahy's (2000) study undermined the patient's right to authenticity and the readers of the signs, having been challenged, emerged afresh as a credible occupational group.

Notes

1   Consultants in the study mentioned 44 different emotions and, on average, each claimed to experience five.

2   In the context of medical negligence, Lavery has argued: 'The response is anger . . . By bringing legal action, the patient also assaults the physician's credibility, insinuating faulty judgement or treatment. Self-esteem and status as a successful practitioner in the community or member of the academic environment are suddenly jeopardized. A malpractice suit challenges professional reliability and authority' (1988: 139).

3   Fears about the greater threat posed by individual grievances have most frequently been discussed in the context of debate about the notion of defensive medicine. This is said to occur when specific procedures, tests or treatment are employed or withheld, expressly for the purpose of averting a possible lawsuit (Ennis and Vincent 1994; see also Ennis et al. 1991; Macfarlane and Chamberlain 1993; Summerton 1995). Bolt (1989) has suggested that

defensive medicine can lead to the doctor-patient relationship shifting from one based on trust to an adversarial one which is totally foreign to everything for which the profession purports to stand, and others have argued that defensive medicine can lead to strategies which can serve to mask errors in clinical medicine (Annandale 1989). Some commentators have suggested that there is little hard evidence that defensive medicine is on the increase (Ham et al. 1988) but despite this, the courts appear to have acknowledged the existence of the phenomenon and many commentators assume this effect. Some judicial pronouncements on the issue suggest that there is something of a crisis in the medical world precipitated by legal intervention into medical decisions. Possibly the best known of these is contained in the judgement of Lord Denning in the classic case of *Whitehouse and Jordan* [1980]: 'Experienced practitioners are known to have refused to treat patients for fear of being accused of negligence. Young men are even deterred from entering the profession because of the risks involved' (658).

4 Positive reactions occur when doctors undertake additional precautionary procedures which might be unnecessary for the proper care of the patient in order to insulate themselves from the possibility of criticism that they had not done everything they could to cure the patient. Negative defensive medicine occurs where treatment which might be justified is withheld because of fears that the risks inherent in treatment might lead to additional harm being caused to the patient.

5 It has also been argued that it may be one factor contributing to the rise in caesarean rates (Macfarlane and Chamberlain 1993). Mulcahy (2000) found that female doctors were much more likely to change at least one aspect of their clinical practice in response to a complaint than were male doctors. Of the 193 male consultants who had had a complaint, 117 (61 per cent) made changes in comparison with 38 (72 per cent) of the 53 females. Where reliable statistics were available, it was shown that men were more likely to engage in fuller consultations with patients and improve their standards of record-keeping. Although a larger percentage of the female practitioners claimed that complaints had had an impact on their medical practice, they were much less likely to implement multiple changes – an average of just one each compared to an average of three alterations each for the male consultants.

6 Consultants in this study were asked whether the way they practised medicine was influenced by the complaints they had received. They were provided with a list of pre-coded responses which drew on the review of literature on defensive medicine conducted by Ennis and Vincent (1994). As with other pre-coded lists, they were given the opportunity to add other responses if they did not appear. The data they provided demonstrate that complaints have a considerable impact on clinical practice.

7 Coates and Penrod (1980–1) and Lloyd-Bostock (1992) have applied this framework to disputes.

8 Sociological studies, based on empirical work in the USA and undertaken in the 1950s and 1960s show how doctors are socialized into these norms of bio-medical culture (Fox 1957; Bucher and Strauss 1960–1; Becker et al. 1961; Stelling and Bucher 1973). Commentators have stressed the importance of experts being able to present authoritative judgements to patients while maintaining an appreciation of the uncertainties of medical science within the medical group. Fox (1957) used the term 'vocabularies of realism' to describe how doctors came to terms with uncertainty. The devices used included emphasis on uncertainties about the course of the disease process in individuals, the limits of clinical knowledge and the practitioner's grasp of this knowledge (Atkinson 1981, 1984, 1995). Bosk (1982) found that technical errors were often tolerated in juniors and Mizrahi (1984) found that coping strategies for distancing and denial were developed by medical interns in relation to such events.

9 Data on the incidence of complaints discussed in Chapter 4 do in fact show that certain specialists were much more likely to have received complaints in the 12 months prior to the study than others. My purpose in revisiting those trends in this chapter is rather different. Here, I am trying to understand the ways in which consultants' interpretation of these trends tends to undermine the status of the complainant.

10 One orthodontic consultant explained: 'There are few downsides to ortho-dontic treatment. It does not involve excessive discomfort and I only feel able to take on patients who really want it done. We only take someone on for treatment if we feel their looks can be improved significantly. In other words, the specialty is designed so that it makes them happy.'

11 Other specialties also have bad news elements. As one obstetrician remarked about obstetrics and gynaecology: 'Sure, we deal with a life-fulfilling event but we also have the opposite. There is the problem of miscarriage which has to be handled sensitively because people see themselves as having lost a child. Other conditions can ruin your sex life or strike at your identity as a woman.'

12 Third parties can also take on the roles of go-betweens or champions for the person criticized (Black and Baumgartner 1983). Third parties of this kind often become embroiled in the dispute and play an active role in it.

13 However, interviews with doctors have also suggested that their willingness to talk about complaints is often related to the content of the complaint and the perceived level of stigma attached to criticism. Thus, there were particular risks attached to discussion of some types of complaint. One doctor in Mulcahy's (2000) study suggested: 'Complaints about sexual impropriety might be difficult to shake off, but complaints about wrong diagnosis or medical care are everyday events'. Others argued that complaints about the unit or lack of funding might be talked about openly, but that those which were more personal were much less likely to surface.

7 Devil and the deep
Mediating differences between doctors and patients

Introduction

Previous chapters have explored the ways in which complaints impact on and mobilize patients and doctors at an individual and collective level. It has been argued that complaints can have a significant and long-lasting impact on medics' and complainants' sense of emotional well-being and can alter the ways in which they experience medicine. But complaints also facilitate a challenge to managers and directors of health services as those ultimately responsible for the quality of service. As public servants guided by legislation laying down clear responsibilities, managers are placed in the difficult position of being expected to consider the interests of service users, colleagues and staff, as well as taking into account the efficient use of hospital resources. For them, the complaints machinery may be called upon to achieve a number of goals which serve managerial needs and at times these will be in conflict with the goals of doctors and complainants. It can, for instance, form part of a public relations exercise, and prevent unfavourable word-of-mouth communications with the service-using community (Gilly et al. 1991; Kadzombe and Coals 1992). Alternatively complaints procedures may act as an early warning system for poor performance and provide valuable data for risk management purposes. Increasing regulation of risk and quality in the NHS provides new incentives for managers to be organizational troubleshooters. 'Modern' managers may be more likely to see complaints positively, as an indication that their organization is approachable and responsive to users' needs, than their medical colleagues. Moreover, the increasing visibility of managers in complaints procedures may well mean that complaints provide an excellent opportunity to regulate medical behaviour under the guise of the rhetoric of patient empowerment.

But the role of managers in complaint handling also reflects a number of tensions. Can they be seen as third parties to disputes who conciliate, mediate, arbitrate and adjudicate, or as minimalist actors who merely facilitate responses? Should they defend staff because they are part of the organization for which the manager is responsible? How do doctors react to managerial interference in complaint handling? Should they defend patients because the service should be geared towards satisfying their needs? Should they protect the state interest? To what extent can they be neutral? These issues are important because they provide insights into the issue of who wields power in the processing of complaints. If managers perform a minimalist role and defer to clinicians, this suggests that, whatever the expectation of the guidance, a self-regulatory model of complaint handling is being reinforced. If managers are playing a more proactive, interventionist role, then the model being adopted is much more akin to the bureaucratic model anticipated by patient groups and policy makers.

The growth of managerial power

It is clear from earlier chapters that recent decades have seen significant increases in managerial power in the NHS. Movement away from a purely self-regulatory medical model has posed a threat to doctors because it has involved a direct diminution of their formal powers. In the years following the creation of the NHS, medics permeated the institutional decision making machinery and represented the voice of authority.[1] Klein (1989) describes, for instance, how in the 1974 reorganization of the service every tier in the administrative hierarchy was festooned with professional advisory committees resulting in the voice of the expert being set 'into the concrete of the institutional structure even more firmly than Bevan had anticipated' (p. 54).[2] In their analysis of the same period Allsop and Mulcahy (1996) draw attention to the assumption in official regulations that senior doctors were their own managers. The 1972 'Grey Book', which catalogued forthcoming administrative changes, explained that the distinguishing feature of the NHS was that in order to do their work properly consultants and GPs *must* have clinical autonomy. It dictated that: 'In ethics and in law they are accountable to their patients for the care they prescribe, and they cannot be held accountable to the NHS authorities for the quality of their clinical judgments so long as they are within the broad limits of acceptable medical practice' (DHSS 1972, para. 1:18).

Successive governments since the late 1970s have aimed to enhance control over the medical profession, especially in relation to spending, and this has been achieved by the gradual introduction of a managerial, as opposed to an administrative, strata. It was the Griffiths Report in 1983 (DHSS 1983a) which finally led to a serious commitment to management of performance and resources. The Report expressed concern about institutional stagnation in the NHS and led to the introduction of general managers at regional, district and hospital level in place of multi-professional teams.[3] Moreover, as

the managerial role became more familiar this new breed of regulators demonstrated an increasing willingness to question the autonomy of doctors. It is no
coincidence that, in the post-Griffiths era, the issue of how to discipline and
dismiss poorly performing doctors was raised much more frequently than had
previously been the case. Moreover, the language and policies of target setting,
review and performance indicators, outcome measures[4] and quality and risk
management heralded a new era in which economists and epidemiologists
have provided managers with tools for questioning and determining medical
decisions which had previously been the jealously guarded domain of the
medical profession.

Policy makers have always spoken of the need for managers and doctors to
work together and involve each other in important decisions but there have
been considerable tensions in such a 'partnership'.[5] Post-Griffiths, managers
had a direct interest in the promotion of change as a result of financial awards
available to them but by way of contrast, the medical profession was more
interested in the preservation of traditional networks of power. In Klein's
words:

> Above all, the medical profession had made sure that governments,
> whatever their ideology or ambitions would think long and hard
> before seeking to change the structure of the NHS in any way which
> would bring the underlying concordat with the medical profession
> into question. From being the main opponents of the NHS, the
> doctors had in effect become the strongest force for the status quo.
>
> (1989: 57)

Tensions have also existed between managers and patients. In the early
years of the NHS it was anticipated that patients' interests were protected by
both managers and doctors who were assumed to represent their individual
and collective needs. A series of high profile reports on mismanaged care in the
1960s and 1970s caused policy makers to be concerned about the willingness
or ability of managers to regulate medical activity in the interests of patients,
and led indirectly to the setting up of CHCs. The introduction of CHCs marked
a recognition that patients' interests were sometimes in direct contrast to
those of managers. This is easily illustrated in relation to complaints which
often relate to resource and policy issues. Moreover, doctors sometimes refer to
a lack of resources as a justification for their behaviour in their responses to
complaints.[6] It is also the case that if a grievance is not resolved to the satisfaction of a complainant, their subsequent appeal may be based on criticisms of
the way the complaints procedure is managed and overseen. It becomes clear
then, that the potential for tension between the needs of patients and doctors
is much more complex than was originally anticipated by the architects of
the NHS.

Challenges to the concordat between profession and state were most evident in the Thatcher era when medics were consistently challenged and made to justify what politicians of the new right came to see as restrictive practices (Perkin 1996). While the NHS before Thatcher's reforms seemed to be highly regulated in practice, the mechanisms to control clinical activity were still weak (Allsop and Mulcahy 1996). The White Paper *Working for Patients* (DoH 1989) and the NHS and Community Care Act 1990 reflected a move to much tighter managerial control of resources and regulation of medical behaviour. For the first time doctors were required to participate in local audits of their work, the allocation of merit awards was reviewed so as to take greater account of both clinical skills and commitment to the management of the service, and doctors were forced to agree job descriptions including the number of hours they spent on NHS work. As though to draw attention to the menacing prospect of tighter regulation, disciplinary procedures were also streamlined.

More recently the establishment of the Commission for Health Audit and Inspection (CHAI) and the National Institute for Clinical Excellence (NICE) have marked a coming of age for performance indicators and spending strategies which are evidence-based and prioritize assessment criteria based on value for money.[7] In the past, managers' attempts to regulate medical work have been hindered by the problem of how non-experts evaluate professional practice. The growth of review and information resources such as NICE, CHAI, the National Patient Safety Agency and the National Clinical Assessment Agency now provide managers with 'objective' criteria according to which the performance of medics can be judged.

The role of managers in handling complaints

The increase in managerial power in the NHS has been reflected in the spirit and wording of successive complaints procedures. Managers have metamorphosed from administrators who serviced the complaint handling needs of doctors towards innovators and regulators. The period from the 1970s to the present has, in particular, seen a shift away from a variety of models towards the development of one set of principles according to which all complaints should be managed, regardless of whether they concern primary or secondary care, doctors or other clinical staff, and clinical or non-clinical issues. Increasing emphasis has also been placed on the independent review of grievance management and the responsibilities of service managers to oversee all complaint handling. Perhaps the best measure of this shift was the fact that the introduction of a new complaints procedure in 1996 brought about the abolition of a separate hospital complaints procedure for handling complaints about clinical care which was designed and managed by doctors. Even before that, the *Citizen's Charter* gave rise to an expectation that all complaints should be seen by the chief executive.[8]

The role of complaints handlers is multi-faceted and there is considerable potential for tension and ambiguity. While managers are expected to oversee formal complaints they are also required to empower front-line staff to deal with complaints on the spot. They are expected to investigate but also to advise and support. There are also differences across sectors which undermine the claim that all complaints are now handled according to the same principles. While there is a requirement that complaints officers in hospital Trusts must be senior managers, complaints officers in general practice are merely required to 'administer' the procedure. Posnett et al.'s (2001) research suggests that those involved with the operation of the procedures are also confused about their role. They found, for instance, that across England, Wales, Scotland and Northern Ireland, 53 per cent of the 359 complaints managers who responded to their survey would like more training on the complaints manager's role and this rose to 70 per cent among Welsh respondents. A further 66 per cent said they would like training on interpreting the regulations.

Despite the fact that the designers of the current procedure purported to have moved away from a system in which there was a separate but parallel clinical complaints procedure, clinicians still exercise a special form of control over clinical complaints. Complaints about family health service practitioners are 'practice owned' and are supposed to be managed entirely from the practice. Health authorities are only empowered to become involved if the practice is not meeting national standards such as those relating to timescales for responses. Moreover, although Trust chief executives are expected to 'sign off' letters of response to formal complaints any response given to a complainant which refers to matters of clinical judgement must be agreed by the clinician concerned or consultant responsible for medical care.[9] No allowance is made for doctors and managers being unable to agree a response. Does this mean that tensions never arise or that policy makers were uncertain how to deal with them?

Knowing what's going on

The formal procedure governing hospital complaint handling anticipates that there will be open channels of communication between staff and managers about complaints. This means that complaints managers are expected to consult the staff involved with the care being complained about. By the same token, front-line staff are expected to refer oral complaints on to the manager responsible for complaint handling where they are sufficiently serious or warrant independent investigation.[10] The distinction between what constitutes an informal and a formal complaint, and the circumstances in which an informal or oral complaint should be referred from service level to a manager or administrator remain ambiguous.[11] Official guidance on the procedure suggests that staff should report these complaints to managers when they are 'serious' or call for a more independent appraisal, but it is local rather than national guidance which governs the criteria according to which staff should determine whether to refer a complaint on. While many complaints are probably well handled at service level in discussions between the person involved and the complainant, there has always been considerable potential in procedures for serious complaints or those involving important quality issues to be hidden from the view of managers. As several commentators on the current procedure have made clear the complaints procedure may be working extremely well but we do not have sufficient data, nor can we feel confident about the data to which we do have access, to be sure that this is the case.

What evidence do we have about the proportion of complaints referred to managers by doctors? Little empirical research has been undertaken in an NHS context which has been concerned with the complaint handling role of managers. Mulcahy's (2000) postal survey of over 400 doctors relates to the pre-1996 procedure although on close scrutiny it would seem that the early stages of both procedures remain depressingly similar. Her data suggest that much activity in response to formal complaints occurs in the shadow of formal procedures.[12] She found that complaints reached consultants through a number of routes. The largest proportion of complaints (40 per cent) was brought to their attention by a manager or administrator but a significant proportion had complaints addressed to themselves or had them referred by medical colleagues,[13] solicitors or a defence union.[14] This placed a third of the consultants complained about in a position to withhold information about criticisms of their behaviour from managers should they choose to do so.

In order to explore what consultants did in response to complaints received, doctors taking part in the postal survey were asked how they had responded to complaints once they had knowledge of them. Regardless of the channel through which the complaint was received, the majority of consultants (60 per cent) attempted to resolve complaints themselves without involving managers. Consultants who responded directly to complainants used a variety of methods for doing so including writing back to the complainant; discussing the matter with the complainant next time they saw them; arranging a specific meeting; or telephoning the complainant. According to doctors, managers coordinated and wrote replies, with the agreement of consultants, in only 20 per cent of cases and were involved in responding to complainants in just over half the cases discussed.

What can managers do about this situation? The emphasis in the formal guidance on service-level handling of grievances and ambiguity about the exact characteristics of complaints serious enough to refer on to managers leaves doctors with a considerable amount of discretion about how to handle complaints. Managers interviewed in Mulcahy's (2000) study were sensitive to the fact that a major implication of complaints not being processed through the formal channels was that an official record could not be kept or the issues raised further investigated. One manager told the story of a retired consultant who left a whole drawer of unanswered complaints in his filing cabinet on his departure, many of them going back years.[15] But even if they did have a range of more precise regulatory powers, research suggests that informal persuasion, reference to the regulatee's and regulator's interests and general standards of morality are more often used to overcome resistance to compliance with rules and regulations than formal sanctions (Baldwin 1990).[16] This is particularly so in the NHS. The implementation of health care policy at local level has always involved managers in persuading and steering doctors. Ham (1992) has argued that since doctors alone tend to determine what is best for their patients, persuasion has traditionally been seen as the most pragmatic approach to rule enforcement. Socio-legal researchers have long argued that interaction with those with whom the 'regulator' is likely to have a long-term relationship is likely to encourage the adoption of an internal and conciliatory stance (Macaulay 1963; Bartrip and Fenn 1980; Hutter 1988; Baldwin 1990). The willingness of managers to enforce formal complaints procedures may be dependent on the size of the hazard identified, the reaction of the responsible party, their past record, the extent to which their decisions were subject to review, the scope of their power, their own moral evaluation of the behaviour, the resources available and the cost of compliance. Somewhat ironically, in his discussion of the willingness to enforce sanctions, Baldwin (1990) argues that the intentions of the regulated have much more impact on enforcement strategy than their level of knowledge about the regulatory framework. It is failure of goodwill, or moral failure, rather than ignorance which is much more likely to prompt a proactive approach to the enforcement of formal legal rules.

Styles of dispute resolution

So far I have focused on the tensions which can arise because of the ways in which complaints procedures continue to reinforce a self-regulatory model of complaint handling at service level. Lack of clarity about when complaints should be referred to managers means that a significant number of complaints appear to be handled in the shadow of the procedures overseen by managers. But what happens when managers are notified of complaints? Do managers and doctors work in partnership or do the tensions apparent at policy level also play themselves out at service level? Little research has been undertaken in this area but Kolb's (1987) work on managers who have a dispute resolution role within organizations is particularly useful in this context. She has described the tensions experienced by 'corporate ombudsmen' employed by organizations to resolve disputes between employees and employers. Role ambivalence of the type discussed above was managed by the ombudsmen in her study by favouring one set of normative expectations over the other – that is, adopting a partisan stance. This manifested itself in one of two ways. First, 'helping' ombudsmen attempted to resolve disputes in a way which satisfied the complainant. They defined their goals as being client satisfaction, usage rates, cost savings and organizational change. Their focus was on the ethics of care, recognition of needs and individualization of solutions. By contrast, the main function of 'fact-finding' ombudsmen was perceived to be containment of the problem for the sake of the organization. These ombudsmen tended to take a more procedural view of their role and to focus on the degree to which organizational policies and procedures were followed. They prioritized 'due process' criteria and placed emphasis on notions of fairness, convenience, consistency and timeliness. In contrast to helping ombudsmen, most of their cases seemed to involve helping the complainant accept disappointment by offering rational explanations for the situations they had complained about. In practice, the distinction between these roles was not as simple it might seem. All the ombudsmen in the study felt the strong draw of organizational demands and the organization's interest in quiet management of the dispute.

Confrontation

A detailed content analysis of questionnaire and interview data with managers (25) and doctors (35) from Mulcahy's (2000) study revealed that two main approaches to complaint handling were also adopted by managers and consultants who had received complaints. These did much to reveal the ideological tensions implicit in a complaints procedure which appears to give both professionals and managers an active role. Unlike the helping and fact-finding roles described above, the first was based on confrontation, with both doctors and managers taking a principled stance against the involvement of the other in managing disputes. A significant group of both consultants and managers argued that the other should be less involved in complaint handling. Of the 35 consultants interviewed, 20 were prompted to give justifications for why they should respond to complainants directly without involving managers. Their responses fall into three categories which can be simply classified as being based on ignorance, ethics and principle. First, a number made it clear that they did not know about the existence of a requirement that they should involve managers in their response to written complaints. Second, some consultants considered it appropriate to respond directly, as a matter of courtesy. They felt that if a complainant had taken the trouble to write to them, then the least they could do was respond personally. Consultants in this group tended to see the allegations as a confidential matter between themselves and the complainant and what was most striking was their appeal to a standard of politeness and to ethical responsibilities. These were presented as professional norms which took precedence over bureaucratic rules. Discussion of the formal procedure was absent from these accounts even though it was obvious from their questionnaire responses that the group was aware of the regulations.[17]

But the third and strongest theme to emerge from the interviews was consultants' outright rejection of the necessity for managerial input in complaint handling. Among this group, managers who sought to coordinate and oversee replies to the complaint were, like the description of complainants in the previous chapter, identified as 'outsiders' who did not possess sufficient medical knowledge to be able to construct a response to a complaint about medical care. This group of 18 of the 35 consultants interviewed felt a direct response was appropriate because the complaint was about a purely clinical issue and were assertive in their claim that managers ought not to be involved in complaints about the standard of care. Consultants justified this reaction by reference to the degree of control they felt they lost when they referred complaints to managers, and the introduction of an unnecessary layer of bureaucracy. To some extent their fear of loss of control was substantiated by other results from the study. Data from questionnaires filled in by doctors revealed that, where the response to the complainant was drafted by an administrator or manager, just under one-third of consultants (62) were not even given an opportunity to approve the response, while 112 (59 per cent) were. In a number of cases consultants claimed that managers also failed to keep doctors informed of the outcome of the complaint and many in the study continued to be concerned about whether the complaint had become a legal claim. The most recent evaluation of the 1996 complaints procedures also found that 50 per cent of NHS staff surveyed were not satisfied with the way they were kept informed of the progress of the complaint. This suggests that channels of communication between managers and doctors continue to be less than perfect (DoH 2001).

In her interviews with managers Mulcahy (2000) found that managers were sensitive to these jurisdictional tensions. A group of just over one-third (9) were just as jealous of their jurisdiction over complaints and as sensitive to possible infringement of their territory as doctors. At one extreme tensions with consultants had reached such a peak that a manager reported having to get advice from the BMA and the Medical Defence Union to prove the scope of his powers under the formal procedure. In the words of another manager, typical of this group: 'Medics never, never accept that anything has ever gone wrong. I don't think the profession should be allowed to investigate their own mistakes. We're all employed by one organization and we should have one method of investigating all complaints'. While maintaining what one interviewee called 'a healthy suspicion of doctors', this group of managers was more likely to be supportive of the complainant's right to voice their grievance and to be empathetic about their concerns. They adopted a confrontational stance against doctors, they also saw themselves in Kolb's guise of a helping ombudsperson as far as complainants were concerned. These managers variously described themselves as a champion or watchdog for consumers, and as being supportive of a proactive approach to complaint handling. As one argued: 'My style is very simple because the complainant is often right. I think we should treat every complainant with respect and sensitivity. They are angry and unhappy about our service and my job is to tell the people who pay for the service the facts.'

These managers justified their active intervention in complaint handling on a number of grounds. The majority stressed that complaint handling was a role which had been formally assigned to them and for which they were accountable. This group focused on jurisdictional tension and was much more prepared to adopt a confrontational approach to doctors who would not cooperate because they saw such activity as a threat to their autonomy. This group argued that the level of regulatory power they had should be seen as commensurate with the amount of responsibility adopted. But practically all the managers interviewed were also keen to stress the place of complaint handling within their quality remit. This group was worried that if they were not involved in handling complaints then complaints could too easily become 'invisible' to the organization.[18] In the words of one manager in Mulcahy's (2000) study:

> When people complain, we should be grateful. They haven't gone to the press, they have taken the trouble to write to us and let us know. But getting that philosophy across is difficult, especially when investigations are inadequately resourced and tend to be something which is tacked on to someone's job. So far, doctors have been so busy reacting that the proactive approach hasn't got a look in.

Managers also justified their increased involvement in complaint handling by reference to the need for impartiality. Such commitment to impartiality varied according to the type of case. Some argued that where fault was found, managers should be prepared to act on their judgement to the detriment of staff within their organization by disciplining them if necessary. For most of the managers in this group, just making a judgement on the merits of a case was considered to be an essential, if difficult, feature of managerial intervention. This approach was thought to be in the interests of both doctors and complainants. These managers echoed the concerns of doctors in the previous chapter when they argued that staff were often not content unless they had an opportunity to exonerate themselves fully from blame by putting their case. Moreover, it was argued that if complaints were to be of use for quality assurance purposes, the validity of particular allegations had to be established. In this sense, the needs of administrative justice reflected the needs of the quality remit. Being distanced from the care relationship or circumstances of the complaint was one way in which managers saw themselves as being able to create a form of impartiality from the parties to the disputes. As one manager explained:

> It's easy to be apologetic about something that has gone wrong when you are not personally involved in it. It's also easier to see the problems with a service when you are not working your guts out every week trying to produce it. Inevitably our staff have an ownership of issues which makes them defensive about complaints. We are here to redress the balance of their inevitably defensive behaviour.

A smaller number of managers in the same study also recognized the importance of facilitating an independent external review of certain complaints. This group had demonstrated its willingness to bring in external agencies to effect the resolution of complaints if necessary.[19] But, such interventions tended to occur only in very serious cases. All senior managers were in agreement that the level of impartiality expected in independent inquiries was a luxury which could not always be justified.

Partnership?

A second group of managers and doctors were less sensitive to jurisdictional tensions and preferred to characterize their relationship as being more akin to a partnership. This group were more like Kolb's fact-finding ombudspersons but the style was much less commonly adopted than the conflictual situations described above, with only one-fifth of respondents regularly handling complaints in this way. Partnerships took a number of different forms. The most common scenario described was for consultants to make a point of talking complaints through with managers in an attempt to deal with the issues raised in them and come to an agreed solution. One of the situations in which consultants had demonstrated their enthusiasm to operate in partnership with managers was when the complaint had the potential to become a legal claim. Such cases were commonly referred to as those warranting the most attention by doctors and managers alike. But, further analysis of data which had originally been placed in the partnership category revealed some partnership arrangements were highly contingent. As one doctor explained:

> Formal complaints are generally dealt with through management. Where a complaint involves clinical judgement then the clinician involved will be asked to respond and I would expect the manager to top and tail his response in line with the clinician's comments. This is

only reasonable. As long as the facts are correct and what they are doing is documenting our opinions, then I think that's fair enough. But if it's about a clinical decision then there is no doubt in my mind that the clinician must respond directly.

In this scenario the partners are not equal. Rather the manager was seen as servicing the consultant's need to make a response to a complaint. Moreover, the 'partnership' arrangement was dependent on the manager allowing the doctor a final veto over the response.

A large proportion of managers interviewed by Mulcahy seemed prepared to take on the minimalist role of junior partner and justify it. Of the 24 managers interviewed, 18 made some form of statement in the course of the interview in support of this vision of the doctor-manager relationship. The adoption of this minimalist stance was a particular feature of interviews with managers who had either a medical or nursing background. Most managers, whether from a clinical background or not, described it as a pragmatic response to lack of effective power, the price to be paid for organizational harmony. Others talked about the long-term costs of pursuing an adversarial strategy with consultants. As one manager put it:

> This medical-profession-versus-the-managers lark doesn't wash with me. I think that the creation of separate tribes and cultures is a right that people should have, but really it's just an excuse by doctors and managers for not taking joint responsibility for the delivery of care. I see some managers who posture a little. They tend to see it as a victory that they have lessened the clinical input into complaint handling. They are out of their depth. But the professional managers see their role as helping things happen in partnership. There is a well of sadism in all of us. We just have to make sure it doesn't leak!

In a similar vein others argued that the adoption of an overly interventionist stance in complaint handling by managers merely resulted in one power elite being replaced by another. As one senior service manager explained: 'You see some managers struggling to topple doctors off their pedestal and all they do is just get up there and keep the space warm for themselves.'

Those adopting this minimalistic approach were also more disparaging of complainants' motives than their interventionist counterparts. The characterizations of complainants by a small subset echoed those made by doctors. Among this group complainants were described as 'deranged', 'petty', having 'nothing better to do' and 'frivolous'. A number described the tactics they employed in an attempt to discourage 'awkward' complaints, including the imposition of time delays on the making of complaints, failure to return calls and referral of complaints to other members of staff. These approaches were often justified by reference to two main arguments. First, that any criticism of a member of staff was also, by implication, a criticism levelled at the services for which the manager was responsible. Second, that complaints can have a detrimental effect on good as well as bad staff. Minimalist managers were also the least likely to see the value of adjudication and were critical of the use of legalistic terminology to describe what, for them, remained a medical issue.

While Mulcahy's (2000) description of managerial styles in complaint handling draws largely on interviews, other research involving a content analysis of complaints files has also suggested that the minimalist approach is common. In their study of hospital complaint files, Mulcahy and Lloyd-Bostock (1994) found little to suggest that managers were carrying out an in-depth investigation of complaints or were at all proactive in complaint handling. In their detailed content analysis of 399 files kept by complaints staff, they found that a total of 422 letters of response were sent to complainants incorporating the organization's account of what had happened. The task of responding to complaints was generally performed by a senior manager with 324 (86 per cent) of responses to complainants coming from a chief executive, assistant chief executive or director of service.[20] Despite the fact that 34 per cent of the complaints in the sample could be classified as involving a clinical element, only 20 (5 per cent) of the officially processed responses to complainants came directly from clinicians. Moreover, managers actively suggested in only 4 per cent of 'investigation cycles'[21] that clinicians respond directly to the complaint. These data suggested that, in practice, the clinical and non-clinical complaints procedures are both overseen by management.[22]

Further analysis of the data by Lloyd-Bostock and Mulcahy (1994) attempted to explore this claim. They found that despite the expectation that complaints handling was the province of chief executives, and that they often signed responses, it was, in reality, delegated to low-level secretarial or administrative staff. But administrative staff to whom complaints were assigned also showed themselves unwilling to accept an active role in complaint handling. The research team originally anticipated that letters to doctors from the officer initiating an investigation cycle would involve a commentary on the complaint made or identify key issues. However, in most cases, 'investigations' consisted of copying the complainant's letter to doctors under cover of a short note asking for a response. Thus, the investigatory stance taken was perfunctory rather than proactive. They found no instances in which either a doctor or complainant was asked for additional details of their account despite the vague nature of many allegations made. Moreover, in 139 (35 per cent) cases, letters of response to complainants incorporated exact passages of text from clinicians' letters of response to the complaint, compiled as part of the investigation cycle. The number of words 'transplanted' in this way ranged from 10 to 840 and in a number of cases included extremely detailed and technical material taken from medical notes. Few attempts were made in these cases at translation of technical or defensive material. It would seem that in over one-third of the files examined officers were little more than a vehicle or 'postbox' through which the counter-arguments of the clinician involved could be expressed (Mulcahy and Lloyd-Bostock 1994).

Recent research suggests a number of reasons why managers continue to be prepared to service doctors in this way. Posnett et al. (2001) found that 41 per cent of the 359[23] hospitals and health authorities which responded to their survey identified their complaints manager as someone who earned less than £24,000 per annum. As 66 per cent of the sample was over 40 years of age, these data suggest that the role is, in reality, still carried out by junior administrators who are not on a career track. Moreover, only 34 per cent of those directly involved in managing complaints reported to the chief executive despite the expectation in the current guidelines that the designated complaints officer should *be* a chief executive or senior manager reporting to the chief executive. The same study found that the majority of complaints managers had responsibilities other than managing complaints and that most commonly this involved legal work (50 per cent) and quality management (19 per cent). The large number of people involved in managing litigation and complaints on behalf of their organization suggests that defence of colleagues is such a regular and vital aspect of their work that a defensive approach to complaint management is likely to be the norm.

Another way to test the willingness of managers to adopt a more proactive approach to complaint handling than has traditionally been expected of them is to look at the extent to which complaints have been used to improve services. Evidence suggests that despite recommendations from various committees and inquiries (DoH 1994, 2000b; Cabinet Office Complaints Task Force 1995a; House of Commons 1999), all of which called for better systems for recording and analysing adverse events, complaints and claims, these systems remain poorly developed. For instance, Kyffin et al. (1997), in an investigation into 12 northern Trusts, found limited recording and monitoring. In the absence of central guidance it was discovered there were different systems in use across Trusts and categories were not broken down to reveal discrete problems that were common across different sources of information. Wallace and Mulcahy (1999) also found that very little action to review service provision was undertaken on completion of an independent review. It would seem that despite the quality rhetoric which abounds in debates about the NHS that events leading to complaints tend to be seen as discrete incidents rather than potential early warnings of systemic failure in integrated information systems. Sadly, a central feature of the reports of the HSC is the oft-repeated concern that the same issues and allegations continue to be raised by complainants.

New roles

Managers have been involved in the handling of complaints about hospitals since the inception of national policies on the matter, but the 1996 complaints procedure introduced a new 'regulator' into complaint handling. It confers responsibility for deciding whether a complaint should be referred to an IRP or a 'convener'. Purportedly, conveners were introduced into the procedure in order to add a greater element of independence in decision making. Official guidance anticipates that the convener will be a non-executive director of a Trust or health authority. This suggests that they are far from being independent but they are not as directly involved in the provision of services as senior managers within the organization. Their remit is also much clearer than the multi-faceted role of managers discussed above. Conveners are required to distance themselves from staff involved in complaints and are expected to ensure that complaints are dealt with impartially at the convening stage. Official guidance makes specific reference to the fact that their function is not to represent either the authority or Trust they are connected with. They are also required to consult with a nominated independent lay panel chair from a regional list in order to prompt a further independent external assessment of the case.[24] Despite these safeguards in the interests of impartiality and independence, are conveners any more likely than managers to adopt a proactive or interventionist stance in complaint handling?

Recent research suggests they are. In determining whether to refer a complaint to an independent panel for further consideration conveners can use one of three powers. They can refer the complaint to an independent panel, reject the case, or send it back for further action by those involved in responding to the complainant at service level. It could be argued that a key indicator of conveners' ability to adopt an impartial stance is their willingness to refer complaints back to staff when they have not been adequately addressed or to call for a panel to be convened. In the first independent evaluation of the 1996 procedure undertaken, Wallace and Mulcahy (1999) found that in a sample of 201 cases described by conveners in a postal survey almost half (47 per cent) had been referred back for further attempts at local resolution and a further 27 per cent were referred on to an independent review for adjudication. When conveners were asked why they thought these problems were occurring they were prepared to openly criticize staff. In doing so they attributed their failings to poor staff training and inexperience in complaint handling (32 per cent). In the words of one convener:

> In a high percentage of cases I have seen I came to the conclusion that the complaint could have been resolved locally had a bit more care and forethought been given to dealing with the complaint. Much of

the formal language used in communications with the complainant makes it appear that they have entered into a structured and fundamentally indifferent system. It is vital that the complainant sees a 'human' as opposed to a bureaucratic organisation. A little sympathy goes a very long way.

Another indication of the willingness of conveners to adopt an impartial stance is who they consult with in coming to a decision as to whether to refer a case on to an IRP. Wallace and Mulcahy (1999) found that Trust conveners commonly approached the complaints team within the hospital or Trust (69 per cent); the trust chief executive (29 per cent); the complainant (20 per cent); the CHC (13 per cent); and much less commonly the staff implicated in the complaint (6 per cent). In contrast, the only other personnel whom the health authority conveners consulted with a frequency of more than 10 per cent was their complaints team (79 per cent). These data suggest that health authority conveners were able to maintain a greater distance than Trust conveners from NHS personnel but are encouraging for consumer groups in that doctors involved do not appear to have been given special treatment over complainants.[25] But, the same study also highlighted concerns that in some organizations the work of the convener was serviced by the very complaints departments against which the complainant had appealed. Concerns about the tensions in the role were not limited to observers. Conveners spoke about the difficulty in distinguishing between investigating the complaint and determining whether it required further investigation. Moreover, the majority (65 per cent) of the 166 lay chairs surveyed, 46 per cent of the 153 Trust conveners and 25 per cent of health authority conveners thought that it was difficult for conveners to be fully independent when they also served as a member of the board of the Trust or health authority involved.[26] Conveners argued that as a non-executive director they worked with many of the senior staff involved in service provision and that this inevitably introduced a bias. A number spoke openly of the natural respect and loyalty they felt for the Trust and acknowledged that this might incline them to give staff the benefit of the doubt. They also argued that as a member of the board they had access to information about the organization and its resources which would not be available to a true outsider and could unduly influence their decision. The anxieties expressed by conveners about the independence of the convening role were widely shared by others including the HSC (HSC 1996–7, 1997–8, 1998–9, 1999–2000, 2000–1). Even when conveners were considered to be doing a balanced assessment there was concern that they did not *appear* to be independent. CHCs' concerns about the real and perceived independence of the convening role are also well documented (ACHCEW 1990) and many of these were reiterated by them in Wallace and Mulcahy's (1999) research.[27]

Conclusion

This chapter has discussed the potential chasm between the formal guidance on hospital complaints and the management of complaints at service level. The focus has been on the use of rules and the meaning attributed to them rather than the rules themselves. The chapter has attempted to place the study of rules within an organizational and social context and suggests that situated power, workload, personality, long-term interests and relationships may have as much impact on the way complaints systems operate as the formal legal framework developed at policy level. Taking such factors into account facilitates what Kahn has described as the 'larger culture of law' (1999: 128). It might be argued that the very idea of the legitimacy of formal rules rests on a model of political power that is rarely realized. The idea of a model in which decisions are made and radiate downwards from the top of a hierarchy appears especially untenable in the NHS where a managerial strata remains a relatively recent innovation and policy makers appear keen to encourage or 'fudge' role ambiguities. The research reviewed suggests that there is much to be learned from empirical studies of how rules operate. Rule circumvention and avoidance may be seen as choices which are just as rational for organizational actors as compliance is. Such reactions to rules are likely to be perceived as deviant by rule makers but competing evaluations are also possible which place the activity within an alternative moral or ethical professional framework. In some cases the effect of rule breaking may be mitigated by the fact that the breach was unintentional or condoned by colleagues. In others, the letter of the law might be preserved by ideas of partnership but the spirit of it is abused.

Despite the intensity of their reactions to allegations about the quality of care they provide, research on the operation of the hospital complaints system suggests that administrators responsible for coordinating the management of complaints do not take a proactive role in conducting investigations and drafting responses. It would seem that the dominance of professional interests – which was apparent in earlier discussions of how the hospital complaints procedure was negotiated – is also reflected at service level. Doctors may be left feeling unsupported but the accounts they provide in response to complaints appear to go unchallenged and there is little evidence of conflict between clinicians and managers when interview accounts are compared with content analysis of complaints files. But there is sufficient evidence that, despite the fact that the majority of managers were content to play a subsidiary role to that of doctors, attitudes are changing. Conflicts of interest clearly exist between managers and consultants, and managers appreciate that they could use data from complaints to help them evaluate services. These conflicts may cause the doctor to question both the legitimacy of managerial complaint

handling and the degree of trust to be afforded managers when handling complaints. The jurisdictional tensions inherent in the formal procedure and day-
to-day interpretation of it are most apparent in the finding that a significant
number of complaints may never come to the attention of managers. This
demonstrates that whatever the intention of policy makers, the effectiveness
of any formal rules is reliant on the extent to which those operating formal
systems embrace the ideologies they reflect. Important interests are at stake in
the debate over who should manage complaints. The tensions revealed reflect
wider changes in the NHS, most notably the increasing moves to place formal
power in the hands of managers and the emergence of hospital-wide programmes such as risk and quality management schemes. These initiatives
assume that doctors should account for their behaviour and require them
to do so. But the differences of opinion between managers and between
managers and doctors reflects ideological and political arguments about
self-regulation which have been rehearsed throughout the history of the NHS.
In the next and final chapter these issues will receive further consideration.

Notes

1 Klein (1989) argues that during this period the real political battle in the
   health care arena was a definitional one. If specific problems could be labelled
   medical then medics claimed jurisdiction over them. The control of spending
   in the first two decades of the NHS provides a good example of the implications of doctors being able to define medical need. During this period, central
   government controlled the budget but clinical teams enjoyed a considerable
   amount of autonomy over spending. At service level it was doctors who made
   decisions about how much treatment patients should get based on their
   assessment of the overriding mandate of medical need. Significantly, neither
   the NHS Act of 1946 nor its successor of 1977 actually defined the nature of
   health, illness and care and what is and what is not the responsibility of the
   state (Salter 1998). The medical imperative of maximizing equipment and
   resources was at odds with budgetary constraints but it was not until the 1970s
   that governments sought to tackle the issue and reclaim what constituted
   appropriate expenditure as a matter to be decided in the political arena.
2 At the time, systems for costing individual items or completed patient episodes
   were lacking. Moreover there was very little data on their effectiveness.
3 During the same period medical and nursing representatives on management
   teams began to lose their veto power.
4 These include such things as mortality rates, studies of postoperative death
   and inquiries into maternal deaths.
5 Although Griffiths envisaged that doctors would become involved in management, the Report was not well received by the profession because it

questioned the ability of doctors alone to determine what was appropriate clinical care and, in the event, few doctors took up managerial posts.

6 Criticisms of resource allocation decisions increasingly feature in medical negligence actions as well.

7 Both these organizations were established to improve the quality of patient care in the NHS but it is the model according to which they do this that provides so much interest in the current context. Both organizations claim to make evidence-based recommendations and both claim to take patient perspectives on care into account. The CHI does this by carrying out clinical governance reviews to ensure that patients' services are improving, patients have all the information they need about their care, health professionals are up to date and clinical errors are prevented wherever possible. In addition, it monitors and reviews how the NHS meets the recommendations of National Service Frameworks and NICE guidelines, and investigates specific service failures. It is significant that the membership of NICE includes not only health professionals but academics and patients.

8 This new approach to complaint handling has come in the wake of an era in which more and more stress is being placed on the regulation of quality and the introduction of risk management. Integrated information systems are crucial to the success of both these initiatives and complaints have been identified as a key performance indicator for NHS managers.

9 The 1996 procedure gives no guidance on what should happen if a manager and medic cannot agree a response. On this point, see the review of the Davies Report in Chapter 4.

10 The requirement for staff to report complaints to managers differs depending on the way it is received and the degree of seriousness. Moreover, it is national rather than local guidance which governs the criteria according to which staff determine whether an oral complaint should be referred on to the complaints officer.

11 In addition, national statistics about hospital complaints are much more detailed than those relating to primary care complaints.

12 This study did not investigate the handling of oral complaints. Because the distinction between formal and informal complaints is often hard to discern the study interrogated hospital consultants about their experiences of responding to written complaints. Oral complaints can also be classified as formal but, in practice, the vast majority of formal complaints are made in writing.

13 Seven per cent fell into this category.

14 Two per cent fell into this category.

15 Many managers in this group were complimentary about the way in which consultants dealt with complaints, preferring to frame their concerns in terms of the 'challenge' of a new culture of complaint handling and managerialism in the NHS. They drew attention to the fact that many of the consultants with

whom they worked had joined the NHS at a time when 'administrators' existed as part of a support service for medical specialties.

16 In many situations, formal rules and sanctions are not referred to directly at all (see Macaulay 1963), although this may be a case of bargaining in the shadow of rules with the *threat* of enforcement underpinning all negotiation (Mnookin and Kornhauser 1979).

17 Official guidance on the hospital complaints procedure (HC(37)88) anticipates that systems for the handling of complaints will be well publicized and made clear to patients and staff. Data from the postal survey of 848 consultants conducted for this book revealed that three-quarters of consultants who had been the subject of a formal clinical complaint were aware of the complaints procedure. One hundred and eighty-nine (77 per cent) respondents said that they were aware of a formal procedure for the handling of complaints in their Trust or unit. However, there were 7 respondents who said that no such procedure existed and 16 did not know one way or the other. Although the majority of consultants knew about the procedure, few had knowledge of its origin or an understanding of its detail. Almost one-quarter of consultants in the complaints sample said that they had no knowledge of who had been responsible for drafting the procedure. The data suggest that the process of negotiating the separation of the clinical complaints procedure remained almost as invisible to rank and file members of the profession as it did to those outside policy making circles. The majority (60 per cent) of consultants thought that the procedure had been designed by health service managers at local (45 per cent), district (9 per cent) or regional (5 per cent) level. Significantly, only 2 per cent mentioned any medical involvement in the drafting of the procedure. There was also a lack of knowledge of the role of the HSC. One hundred and twenty-five (51 per cent) consultants said that they did not know what this role entailed. By contrast, all the managers interviewed had a detailed knowledge of the procedure. Interviews revealed a common process for dealing with complaints which involved written enquiries being made to members of staff who were either mentioned in the complaint or who worked in, or supervised, the department being criticized. The person contacted tended to be a head of department or a clinical consultant approached in his or her managerial capacity. Any one complaint might involve several issues and thus generate several enquiries.

18 Some managers had a complaints group specifically responsible for discussing the lessons which could be learned from complaints and almost all the managers interviewed ensured that their board received a quarterly memorandum which outlined the number of complaints received, the timescale taken to deal with them and some details of the issues raised. One unit was in the process of setting up a review body which would have the responsibility to comment on the tone and content of responses.

19 Two managers in the study had introduced a scheme whereby clinical

complaints about specialties with few representatives in that hospital were referred to an independent clinical specialist for review. The results of the review were made available to both the complainant and the clinician complained about. Another manager had used his powers, on several occasions, to order an independent inquiry into cases which had been taken up by the media and which he felt were so serious that no one within the hospital would be seen as being impartial enough to handle them fairly.

20   A further 39 (9 per cent) came from directors of services or the head of administrative services and 8 (2 per cent) from either the chair of the health authority, district general manager or district medical officer.

21   These included letters sent from managers or administrators to those named in the complaint and responses to them.

22   The discrepancy between this study and Mulcahy's later study is probably best understood as a reflection of the fact that Mulcahy's study related to all written complaints received by doctors while Mulcahy and Lloyd-Bostock's content analysis of complaints involved complaints which had reached the formal complaints procedure and come to the attention of managers.

23   This number constitutes 69 per cent of Trusts and health authority/boards in the UK.

24   However, the procedure makes it clear that ultimately it is for the convener to decide whether or not to set up a panel (NHSE 1996).

25   There was some debate among participants in the survey as to whether an approach to a complainant was appropriate. This suggested some role ambivalence or ambiguity. Some conveners reported that they had been positively advised against speaking to the complainant so as not to compromise their impartiality. Others felt it was reasonable to do so in order to keep them informed of progress and seek clarification.

26   The authors suggest that the difference in views between health authority and Trust conveners can be explained by the fact that in the majority of cases health authority conveners assess complaints about GP services for which they bear no direct responsibility.

27   A number of instances of poor practice were cited including conveners being protective of Trusts and trying to avoid panel hearings, and conveners failing to consult independent chairs or clinical assessors as required.

8 A new hope
Concluding thoughts

Introduction

The aim of this book has been to examine the ways in which the needs of doctors, complainants and the state have been conceptualized by policy makers and are played out in everyday contexts. It has sought to explore one aspect of the interface between the state, the individual and powerful professional groups in society and has much to say about the impact of formal law in regulating such relationships. Most importantly, it has provided an opportunity to examine how a form of regulation negotiated by policy makers and elite groups at national level operates, and is constantly renegotiated, at service level. When looking at the connections between these two levels the book has sought to emphasize the general continuities between the legal system of formal rules and the social system of which it forms a part. In this final chapter, I will reflect upon the main themes to emerge from the studies reported in earlier chapters, and their wider implications.

The study of complaints has been marginalized by public lawyers, sociologists and social policy analysts alike. Complaints have been both under-researched and under-theorized. This is surprising given that the study of disputes raises important issues for social scientists and lawyers. In particular, previous chapters have suggested how complaining prompts the construction and reconstruction of moral, ethical and disputing identities. It would seem, then, that the study of low-level disputes has considerable potential to bring the sociological imagination of macro-level abstract theories to bear on the mundane drama of everyday life. But to date, complaints have not been viewed as involving matters of principle or sufficiently serious grievances to warrant intensive study. Academic and public debate has tended to emphasize the dominant role of the courts, tribunals and ombudspeople in discussions of accountability and access to justice. In truth, the basis for judicial intervention in public administration is so narrow and adjudication by the courts and many tribunals so rarely sought that such contentions are ripe for challenge. This book has attempted to redress such imbalance and to make the case for the study of complaints to occupy a more central role in socio-legal scholarship. It has sought to draw attention to the various ways in which the parameters of legitimate public activity are constantly being reconfigured away from the gaze of the formal legal system. Low-level systems of grievance resolution provide processes through which public sector officials and professional groups can be held accountable for their activity.

The need for effective complaints procedures is particularly critical in the public sector. These services are often in a monopoly position and the option of exiting a service is rarely available for users. Considerable inequalities of bargaining power between service provider and service user are the norm and these are further exacerbated when a service based on particular expertise is being provided, as is the case in the NHS. Many public services are provided for those who are among the most vulnerable, frail and disadvantaged members of our society. These are often the very people who do not have the resources to access more complex and expensive systems for redress, such as the courts. For many, complaints systems are the first and only part of the civil justice system they will use. Most importantly, many more people will use these systems than will use courts and tribunals. It is in these service-level interactions, rather than the high profile cases which hit the headlines, that the tensions between individuals, powerful groups and the state are most commonly played out.

The medical profession has played an extensive role in determining how doctors can be challenged and the aspects of their work which can be subjected to review. Early models of complaints procedures relied heavily on the principle of self-regulation, which privileged professional narratives, and the profession continues to play a key role in policing the regulatory boundaries set by the state. For many this has been an acceptable state of affairs in which experts are treated with the respect which their dedication and long training calls for. Self-regulation has been particularly attractive to the state as it has allowed successive governments to hive off responsibility for overseeing the competence of medical work. But relations between the state, the profession and the citizenry are in a constant state of flux and the symbiotic relationship between state and profession has increasingly become a cause for concern among those who consider it the state's role to question the position of powerful groups in society. Each new version of complaints procedures introduced since the birth of the NHS has demonstrated that the notion of accountability is both culturally specific and time sensitive. As consumer groups have become organized and vocal, complaints systems have become more focused on a legal-bureaucratic model of justice which assumes that the parties to a dispute have equally valid narratives. The patient expects, and is increasingly supported in their claim to be able to demand, a reasoned response. It is anticipated by the state, the legal profession and patient groups that doctors should have to justify their behaviour. In so doing, they may well be called upon to articulate what is involved in their expert work and answer questions different from those usually posed. This shift to a rights-based culture has served to threaten the delicate balance between state regulation, clinical autonomy and managerial or consumer interference in medical work. In turn, these issues touch upon even more fundamental moral panics in our society about the ways in which a discourse of rights displaces ideologies of trust and harmony.

Complaints by patients and their relatives represent a disruption of the ceremonial order of the medical encounter, but the dominance of scientific discourse has made it hard for patient accounts of health and illness to be given the same level of legitimacy as those provided by doctors. The well of frustration this creates for patients who wish to enjoy autonomy becomes particularly obvious when complaints are made. When patients call doctors to account they step out of the 'sick role' anticipated of them. Complaints call into question the doctor's technical and moral authority and require that their traditional roles be renegotiated. Patients' common-sense accounts of illness and treatment contain explicit and implicit challenges to the bio-medical accounts of doctors and suggest that patients also possess a unique under-standing of health and illness. They represent a threat to the objectivity of expert knowledge and question the impartiality of that knowledge. These signs of dissent become even more explicit in complaints which can be seen as sites of resistance to the imbalance of power in the doctor-patient relationship, and as claims to alternative ways of knowing.

It becomes clear then that the challenge of complaints goes well beyond individual grievances and responses to them. They are also symbols of the larger threat of consumerism and the legitimation of lay narratives. But there is another thread to the symbolic challenge of complaints which is likely to cause even more disruption to dominant models of the doctor-patient rela-tionship. Studies of the incidence of medical mishap and dissatisfaction have begun to make clear that voiced grievances are but the tip of the iceberg. Many complaints chronicle perceptions that there has been a medical mishap. Some are substantiated, others are not. But these new studies of mishap, many of which have been undertaken by doctors, demonstrate that the vast majority of errors are not acted upon by patients and their relatives. Most importantly they are not always acted upon by the doctors at service level who are best equipped to identify the mistakes caused by others. If the medical profession are unable to respond to the challenges posed by risk and quality management systems then complaints are bound to be accorded prime importance as an external safety valve. Some complaints may be misplaced criticisms of tech-nical care but they provide a trigger for managerial interference. The challenge posed here is not one of alternative discourses but exposure of the failures of the profession to manage quality of care and poor performance.

Accountability is particularly important in the medical sphere because of the consequences of error for patients and doctors. The vast majority of doctors work hard to alleviate pain and reduce the harmful consequences of illness and disease. Like everyone else they make mistakes. Some doctors make mistakes on a regular enough basis to be labelled incompetent by their peers and patients. But not all medical mistakes are caused by incompetent doctors. Discrete mistakes are made by doctors who are otherwise extremely capable and diligent. These mistakes occur because of fatigue, a temporary lapse of concentration, lack of understanding and misjudgement. They may also occur because a 'slip' which seems inconsequential may contribute to a major error because of a whole chain of events in the control of different members of a clinical team. What marks medical mistakes out from many other mistakes made in the workplace is that they can have fatal consequences. Last week, when grading a postgraduate's essay, I inserted the wrong grade on the mark sheet. I might never had noticed if a diligent colleague had not queried a low mark for a student who is among the best of her cohort. Before I had time to correct the mistake I had probably lost a little of my colleague's respect and upset the student in question. It took me a couple of minutes to change the mark and ten minutes to apologize to the student. If I had been a doctor, a comparable clerical error could have led to someone being administered the wrong dosage of a drug and caused their death.

If asked to prioritize whose needs should be privileged in complaint handling and future reform of complaints systems, I would argue that it is service users whose needs and interests are most in need of protection. This was a fundamental objective of the political architects of the NHS, although it has proved much harder to implement than to plan. Users of health services continue to have little situational power and usually make complaints at a time when they are ill or hurting. When they voice their grievances about medical care, complainants are challenging a huge and organized organ of the state as well as a powerful professional group. Their decision to complain is not taken lightly and many complainants fear retribution. The research reported in this book indicates that the handling of their grievance by managers and doctors can also serve to exacerbate their feelings of hurt and distrust, and can leave their sense of grievance languishing long after the formal process of responding to it has been completed.

Successive studies have demonstrated that a natural reaction to being called to account is to provide a defence. But tragically for complainants defences are framed in ways which undermine the validity of the very act of complaining. This is particularly the case in Anglo-American inspired models of justice where adversariality is positively encouraged. Data presented in this book show that doctors' reconstruction of a valuable sense of identity relies on a deconstruction and undermining of both the complaint and the complainant. Doctors strive to emphasize their different explanations of the cause of events complained about. In contrast to the shared decision making models referred to above, patients are commonly allocated the more traditional roles of difficult, irrational or unknowing subjects in comparison with the rational and knowing doctor. In this professional identity work, doctors seek to externalize blame, maintain the image of the competent expert-knowledge worker and feel justified in making assertions about the superiority of their form of narrative. Doctors' claim to expertise is based on the notion that medicine is a scientific and rational exercise. This allows them to argue that they can approach patients, the objects of their experience, with the purity of an unprejudiced gaze. This is particularly problematic in the context of complaints because such professional judgements are, even if possible, likely to become clouded by the intense emotional reactions to being challenged.[1]

But these findings should not mean that consideration should not also be given to the difficulties experienced by doctors in coming to terms with complaints. The data presented in this book also make it clear that complaints prompt a severe, and often long-lasting, emotional reaction. Doctors argue that they are often the victims of unreasonable and improper demands and they too experience feelings of powerlessness and vulnerability. The emotional responses of doctors to complaints are not those generally associated with members of powerful elites. The strength of their response suggests that complaints can cause a temporary loss of confidence and a legitimation crisis. Why is this so? The making of a complaint challenges the core assumption that health care professionals heal and alleviate pain. For those who see the practice of medicine as their vocation, this can upset constructions of self-identity. Basic tenets of the relationship between patients and doctors are called into question and can lead to a breach of trust, suspicion and anger.

I have argued, along with others, that these intense reactions to complaints have to be understood within the context of the perfectibility model to which doctors aspire in the course of their education. It is clear that medical educators have largely failed, and continue to fail, doctors when they socialize them to strive for error-free practice. Courses on communication skills and doctor-patient interactions are all too often marginalized within medical education and programmes which focus on law and medical ethics tend towards philosophical debate rather than the practical realities of everyday challenges. The elite of the profession have been slow to accept the suggestion that medical care is more than good technical care and that communicating well means more than imparting information. Improvements are being made. Professionals in the primary care sector have demonstrated much more of a propensity than their secondary care counterparts to consider these issues. The debate which has arisen around the value of patient narratives is particularly stimulating. But there continues to be considerable scope for elite professional groups to promote and validate such discussions. This subject alone warrants another book but I see it as no coincidence that these debates about what might be labelled the 'feminization' of medical education are occurring in those sectors of the health service which operate furthest away from medical elites in the Royal Colleges and medical schools. Let us hope that those radicals who today argue in favour of shared decision making are tomorrow's conservatives.

But, for now, considerably more attention needs to be given to supporting doctors in coping with the aftermath of mishaps, complaints and legal claims. Whatever the rights and wrongs of respective positions, complaints draw attention to the ways in which the patient and doctor are motivated to attend to different aspects of 'shared' experiences which result in different qualitative meanings being attached to their encounters. While the doctor is trained to perceive illness as a collection of physical signs and symptoms which define a particular disease state, the patient focuses on the impact of the illness on their everyday life. The encounters recorded in this book suggest that there is a systemic distortion of meaning in doctor-patient disputes which results from the fact that doctors and patients continue to experience illness and disease in significantly different ways.

Again, in considering the threat posed by complaints, it is clear that their significance goes way beyond their impact on the individual. Studies of complaints reveal how they mobilize medical networks and turn the reconstruction of medical identity into a group activity. In their attempts to come to terms with challenges to their expertise, doctors draw on collective understandings of the nature of medical work which allow them to reassert the importance of scientific rationality and expertise. It is with the support of medical colleagues that they come to understand complaints in the context of traditional models of illness and, at times, as a manifestation of disease. This allows them to explain complaints by reference to a bio-medical model which positions the doctor as the giver of the diagnosis and observer of signs. The extensive use of support networks is suggestive of the ways in which the medical fraternity plays a part in the day-to-day responses to complaints made by individual doctors. The dominance of the medical collective is reinforced by the fact that so few consultants seek help from people outside it.

Data presented in this book have revealed that the threat of outside interference also exists in relation to managerial handling of complaints. For some, the initial threat posed by a patient complaint is exacerbated by the opportunity it gives managers to question and attempt to oversee medical work and set boundaries around what is considered appropriate behaviour. In this context, complaints prompt discussion about the degree of accountability that doctors owe to patients, managers and the state. Both doctors and managers are sensitive to the jurisdictional tensions posed by the formal complaints system. It is also apparent that managers and consultants react to these 'turf wars' in very different ways. Doctors are concerned that managers do not have sufficient interest in the protection of medical reputations and that their interest in handling complaints is to adopt an overly conciliatory stance with complainants. Managers are concerned that the tendency of some doctors to react defensively to complaints can cause an escalation of issues and that under-reporting of complaints means that the quality issues raised by complaints can never be fully considered. Some are adversarial and go to considerable lengths to assert their formal or moral authority over complaint handling, while others act in partnership with their medical colleagues. Whichever approach is adopted, doctors have shown themselves willing to react by flouting bureaucratic rules. Such avoidance is often justified by reference to opposing normative frameworks, in particular the ethical standards imposed by the profession. As expert workers with high social standing and significant levels of control over their own work, doctors are well placed to resist the degradation and compulsion which they see managers as routinely attempting to inflict on them. The number of complaints which remain hidden from managers emphasizes the built-in constraints on the capacity of organizations, and governments, to impose their rules on unwilling participants. Such resistance is an important expression of selfhood and collective power. In this way, it can be seen that complaints provide opportunities for mundane and everyday resistances to being called to account by outsiders which are supported by collective ideals.

What next?

What are the implications of the research reported here? In Chapter 1, I argued that policy initiatives, such as increasing attempts to regulate complaint handling, can only be realistic if we improve our understanding of how people using and providing services respond to the broad range of threats posed to the integrity of the professional group. The issue of how social power is wielded by professionals at service level and challenged in complaints is central to identifying how social policy is most likely to be effective and responsive regulation achieved. This book has drawn attention to the many ways in which doctors have resisted regulation of their work. Their resistance has taken many forms and operated at many levels. Some of these have been more visible than others. They have challenged formal bureaucratic controls on their autonomy in national debate, they have promoted the development of self-regulatory models of complaint which emphasize the supremacy of medical knowledge over other understandings of health and illness. Other forms of resistance to being regulated have been less obvious and less well researched. This book has shown how resistance is also an everyday activity of those treating patients and that it goes on in local hospitals as well as on the national stage.

The studies discussed reveal much about the difficulties of integrating bureaucratic and professional models in the provision of public services. Discussion of how professional groups can be integrated within bureaucratic structures is not new. In the NHS, doctors are an active and important force in determining the ways in which services are provided and professional workers held to account. As Hunter has suggested:

> Ministers think they have doctors on the run as they turn up the heat under the General Medical Council and the Royal Colleges in the aftermath of several celebrated cases of malpractice or worse . . . If the government truly wishes to redesign the NHS, then it needs to adopt a radically different prescription and model of change management that appreciates the distinctive features and seeks to work with doctors not against them.
>
> (2000: 18)

But the situation is not as simple as taking the needs of doctors into account. It is undoubtedly the case that the NHS remains highly fragmented in its culture, and that several sets of values compete for supremacy. It is, at best, a coalition of vested interests and it may only be through a process of negotiated order that reforms of the kind discussed in this chapter will succeed. It also remains the case that there continue to be many different models of regulation and each rests on a different ideological foundation. But, the policy environment is changing rapidly and there are many indications that debate on complaints will become one of the areas where tensions between policy makers, the profession, managers and patients will be played out.

There are also signs that the public is less sympathetic to the needs of hospital doctors than was once the case. Debates about the most appropriate form of regulation and concerns about the effectiveness of self-regulation are becoming increasingly common. The inquiries into the murder of patients by Harold Shipman, the handling of poor practice at the Bristol Royal Infirmary and concerns about the irregularities in smear testing at Kent and Canterbury Hospital have all brought concerns about the safety of patients to the fore.[2] In parallel with these developments, the DoH has launched a raft of initiatives aimed at encouraging a more systemic approach to the identification of quality issues, including most notably the setting up of CHAI, CHI, NICE, NPSA and NCAA. These developments have led to the proliferation of clinical protocols which seek to regularize the practice of clinical work. In turn, these have provided a policy environment in which more radical renegotiation of the compact between the state and the profession can take place.

Since coming to power in 1997, the Labour government has laid stress on achieving higher standards in health care; better and more equal outcomes from health care interventions; greater partnership with patients; greater accountability; and the undermining of elites. Complaints also remain on the agenda. New policy objectives will be achieved within the context of a stricter regulatory regime designed for early identification of poor practice by professionals or managers, and it has been widely accepted in policy circles that complaints have an important part to play in such systemic approaches to quality. In 1999, the Cabinet Office Service First Unit published new guidance on how to deal with public sector complaints and the complaints system introduced in 1996 has been formally evaluated and been reformed. There is a commitment to 'modernizing' the NHS and proposals to improve quality are set out in *The New NHS* (DoH 1997) and *A First Class Service* (DoH 1998). In future, the monitoring of both the content and handling of complaints is likely to play a part in reviews carried out as part of clinical audit and clinical governance within health authorities, Trusts and primary care groups as well as the reviews undertaken by the CHI. In addition, professional bodies have introduced important changes which increase the amount and extent of self-regulation. Most notably, the GMC has brought in measures to improve the standards of doctors who have been identified as performing poorly. There is also a new scheme for regular revalidation of practising doctors (GMC 1998).

But there are also signs of tensions between elite medical groups with an interest in regulation as the BMA's vote of no-confidence in the GMC following the publication of the Ritchie Report on Rodney Ledwerd suggests (DoH 2000a; Moore 2000). We are still dogged by a system for educating doctors which leaves them unprepared to deal with being called to account. We continue to be dominated by notions of justice which focus on placing blame on individuals despite the wealth of evidence that the vast majority of medical mishap is caused by systemic error. Most importantly, we are subjected to regular reports of how medical mishap has been covered up and patient concerns about the quality of care marginalized. Is there new hope? Of course. The greater the demand for accountability and the greater the move towards a coherent web of regulatory frameworks, the louder are the calls for changes to the organization of medicine in the interests of both doctors and patients. The challenges to medical work posed by complaints are both an antecedent to, and a reflection of, changes in societal attitudes towards doctors. It can only be hoped that in the future they will become a more effective tool for improving the responsiveness of the medical elite and opening up debate about the validity of the different voices to be heard in the medical encounter.

Notes

1   It has been suggested that the emergence of scientific rationality has allowed modern medicine to promote a different vision of illness from that which went before. Foucault (1973) has argued that, for medical experience to become possible as a form of knowledge, it has been necessary for hospitals to

become organized, for a special status to be developed for the patient, for the state to enter into partnership with the medical profession and for a certain relationship between help and knowledge to be developed. In short, that patients have to be enveloped in a collective homogenous space. The impact of this is that the disease and diagnosis is substituted for the person being treated. The ways in which medical work is organized provide conditions for work shelter in which the collective identity of doctors as ethical, conscientious, competent and stable is maintained.

2   See, for example, *British Medical Journal* (1998); *Daily Telegraph* (1998); House of Commons (1999).

References

ACHCEW (Association of Community Health Councils for England and Wales) (1990) *The NHS Complaint Procedure: ACHCEW's Memorandum to the Public Administration Committee*. London: ACHCEW.

Ackroyd, E. (1986) The patient's complaint, *British Journal of Hospital Medicine*, December: 454.

Allsop, J. (1994) Two sides to every story: complainants' and doctors' perspectives in disputes about medical care in a general practice setting, *Law and Policy*, 16(2): 149–84.

Allsop, J. (1995) *Health Policy and the NHS: Towards 2000*. London: Longman.

Allsop, J. (1998) Complaints and disputes in the family practitioner committee setting 1976–86. Unpublished PhD thesis, University of London.

Allsop, J. (2001) A form of haunting. Unpublished conference paper.

Allsop, J. and Mulcahy, L. (1996) *Regulating Medical Work – Formal and Informal Controls*. Buckingham: Open University Press.

Allsop, J. and Mulcahy, L. (1998) Maintaining professional identity: doctors' responses to complaints, *Sociology of Health and Illness*, 20(6): 802–24.

Allsop, J. and Mulcahy, L. (1999) Reconstructing medical identities, in M. Rosenthal, L. Mulcahy and S. Lloyd-Bostock (eds) *Medical Mishaps: Pieces of the Puzzle*. Buckingham: Open University Press.

Allsop, J. and Mulcahy, L. (2000) Dealing with clinical complaints, in C. Vincent and R. Clements (eds) *Managing Risk in the NHS*, 2nd edn. London. BMA Publications.

Andreasen, A. (1985) Consumer responses to dissatisfaction in loose monopolies, *Journal of Consumer Research*, 12: 135–41.

Andrews, L., Stocking, C., Krizek, T. et al. (1997) An alternative strategy for studying adverse events in medical care, *The Lancet*, 349: 300–4.

Annandale, E. (1989) The malpractice crisis and the doctor-patient relationship, *Sociology of Health and Illness*, 11(1): 1–23.

Annandale, E. and Hunt, K. (1998) Accounts of disagreements with doctors, *Social Science and Medicine*, 1: 119–29.

Arksey, H. (1994) Expert and lay participation in the construction of medical knowledge, *Sociology of Health and Illness*, 16(4): 448–68.

Atkinson, P. (1981) *The Clinical Experience: The Construction and Reconstruction of Medical Reality*. Farnborough: Gower.

Atkinson, P. (1984) Training for certainty, *Social Science and Medicine*, 19: 949–56.

Atkinson, P. (1995) *Medical Talk and Medical Work*. London: Sage.

Audit Commission (1993) *What Seems to be the Matter? Communication Between Hospitals and Patients.* London: HMSO.

Ayuzawa, J. (2001) Efforts to prevent adverse events in the United States – health care risk management and a fresh perspective on adverse events prevention, *Japanese Journal of Cancer and Chemotherapy*, 28(3): 290–303.

Baldwin, R. (1990) Why rules don't work, *Modern Law Review*, 53(3): 321–37.

Bartrip, P. and Fenn, P. (1980) The administration of safety: the enforcement policy of the early factory inspectorate 1844–64, *Public Administration*, 58: 87–102.

Bates, D.W. (2000) Using information technology to reduce rates of medication errors in hospitals, *British Medical Journal*, 320: 788–91.

Bates, D.W., Makary, M.A. and Brennan, T.A. (1998) Information management: asking residents about adverse events in a computerized dialogue: how accurate are they? *The Joint Commission Journal on Quality and Improvement*, 24: 197.

Becker, H., Geer, B., Hughes, E. and Strauss, A. (1961) *Boys in White: Student Culture in Medical School.* Chicago: University of Chicago Press.

Belant, J. (1975) *Professions and Monopoly: A Study of Medicine in the United States and Great Britain.* Berkeley, CA: University of California Press.

Ben-Sira, Z. (1976) The function of the professional's affective behaviour in client satisfaction: a revised approach to social interaction theory, *Journal of Health and Social Behaviour*, 17: 2–11.

Beran, R.G. (2001) Ethical dilemmas of potential adverse events, *Medicine and Law*, 20(3): 385–92.

Berwick, D., Enthoven, A. and Bunker, J. (1992a) Quality management in the NHS: the doctor's role I, *British Medical Journal*, 304: 53–6.

Berwick, D., Enthoven, A. and Bunker, J. (1992b) Quality management in the NHS: the doctor's role II, *British Medical Journal*, 304: 304–8.

Birkinshaw, P. (1985a) *Grievances, Remedies and the State.* London: Sweet & Maxwell.

Birkinshaw, P. (1985b) Departments of state, citizens and the internal resolution of grievances, *Civil Justice Quarterly*, 4: 15–48.

Black, D. and Baumgartner, M. (1983) Toward a theory of the third party, in K. Boyum and L. Mather (eds), *Empirical Theories about Courts.* New York: Longman.

Blaxter, M. (1983) The cause of disease: women talking, *Social Science and Medicine*, 17: 56–9.

Bolt, D. (1989) No-fault compensation – the BMA proposals, in R. Mann and J. Harvard (eds), *No-fault Compensation in Medicine.* London: Royal Society of Medicine Services Limited.

Boreham, N.C., Shea, C.E. and Mackway-Jones, K. (2000) Clinical risk and collective competence in the hospital emergency department in the UK, *Social Science and Medicine*, 51(1): 83–91.

Bosk, C. (1979) *Forgive and Remember: Managing Medical Failure* (1st edn). Chicago: Chicago University Press.

Bosk, C. (1982) *Forgive and Remember: Managing Medical Failure* (2nd edn). Chicago: Chicago University Press.

Bovbjerg, R. et al. (1997) Administrative performance of no-fault compensation for medical injury, *Law and Contemporary Problems*, 60: 71–102.

Brazier, M. (1987) *Medicine, Patients and the Law*. Harmondsworth: Penguin.

Brennan, T., Leape, L., Laird, N. et al. (1991) Incidence of adverse events and negligence in hospitalised patients: the results from the Harvard Medical Malpractice Study I, *New England Journal of Medicine*, 324: 370–6.

Bristol Inquiry (2001) *Report of the Public Inquiry into Children's Heart Surgery at Bristol Royal Infirmary 1984–95*. London: Stationery Office.

British Medical Journal (1998) Children undergoing heart surgery at the Bristol Royal Infirmary, *British Medical Journal*, 316: 1924.

Brook, R.H., Berg, M. and Schecter, P.A. (1973) Effectiveness of non-emergency care via an emergency room, *Annals Intern. Med.*, 78: 333–9.

Brown, H. and Simanowitz, A. (1995) Alternative dispute resolution and mediation, in C. Vincent (ed.) *Clinical Risk Management*, London: BMJ Books.

Bucher, R. and Strauss, A. (1960–1) Profession in process, *American Journal of Sociology*, 66: 325–34.

Cabinet Office (1988) *Improving Management in Government: The Next Steps*. London: Cabinet Office.

Cabinet Office Complaints Task Force (1993a) *Effective Complaints Systems: Principles and Checklist*. London: HMSO.

Cabinet Office Complaints Task Force (1993b) *Speed and Simplicity*, Discussion Paper 2. London: HMSO.

Cabinet Office Complaints Task Force (1994a) *Access*, Discussion Paper 1. London: HMSO.

Cabinet Office Complaints Task Force (1994b) *Fairness*, Discussion Paper 3. London: HMSO.

Cabinet Office Complaints Task Force (1994c) *Attitude and Motivation*, Discussion Paper 4. London: HMSO.

Cabinet Office Complaints Task Force (1994d) *Information*, Discussion Paper 5. London: HMSO.

Cabinet Office Complaints Task Force (1994e) *Interim Report*. London: HMSO.

Cabinet Office Complaints Task Force (1995a) *Putting Things Right*, Main Report, London: HMSO.

Cabinet Office Complaints Task Force (1995b) *Complaint Handling: A Good Practice Guide*. London: HMSO.

Cabinet Office Complaints Task Force (1995c) *Complaints: Literature Review*. London: HMSO.

Cabinet Office Complaints Task Force (1995d) *Complaint Handling in the Public Sector*. London: HMSO.

Cabinet Office Service First Unit (1999) *The Good Practice Guide*. London: HMSO.

Caplan, P. (1995) Anthropology and the study of disputes, in P. Caplan (ed.) *Understanding Disputes: The Politics of Argument.* Oxford: Berg.

Carmel, S. (1988) Hospital patients' responses to dissatisfaction, *Sociology of Health and Illness,* 10(3): 262–81.

Carrier, J. and Kendall, I. (1990) *Medical Negligence: Complaints and Compensation.* Aldershot: Avebury.

Cartwright, F. (1977) *The Social History of Medicine.* London: Longman.

Cassell, E. (1991) *The Nature of Suffering and the Goals of Medicine:* Oxford: Clarendon Press.

Castle, B. (1980) *The Castle Diaries 1974–1976.* London: Weidenfeld & Nicolson.

Catto, G (2002) Change needed after turbulent years, *GMC News,* 11 April.

Chalcroft, S. (2001) Adverse events in hospitals, *New Zealand Medical Journal,* 114(1124): 21.

Charles, S.C. (1984) A different view of malpractice, *Chicago Medicine,* 87: 338–42.

Charles, S.C. and Kennedy, E. (1988) *Defendant: A Psychiatrist on Trial for Medical Malpractice.* New York: Free Press.

CHI (Commission for Health Improvement) (2001) *Investigation into Issues Arising from the Case of Loughborough GP Peter Green.* London: CHI.

Christakis, N. (1999) *Death Foretold: Prophecy and Prognosis in Medical Care.* Chicago: University of Chicago Press.

Citizen's Charter Unit (1991) *The Citizen's Charter: Raising the Standard,* Cm. 1599. London: HMSO.

Coates, D. and Penrod, S. (1980–1) Social psychology and the emergence of disputes, *Law and Society Review,* 15(3–4): 655–80.

Cohen, A. (1994) *Self-Consciousness: An Alternative Anthropology of Identity.* London: Routledge.

Cornwall, J. (1984) *Hard Earned Lives.* London: Tavistock.

Coyle, J. (1999) Exploring the meaning of 'dissatisfaction' with health care: the importance of 'personal identity threat', *Sociology of Health and Illness,* 21(1): 95–123.

Craig, P. (1994) *Administrative Law.* London: Sweet & Maxwell.

Crossman, R. (1972) *A Particular View of Health Service Planning.* Glasgow: University of Glasgow Press.

Crossman, R. (1977) *The Diaries of a Cabinet Minister: Volume 3 1968–1970.* London: Hamish Hamilton.

Daily Telegraph (1998) Problems with examinations of cervical smears at Kent and Canterbury Hospital, *Daily Telegraph,* 31 January.

Danzon, P.M. (1985) *Medical Malpractice – Theory, Evidence, and Public Policy.* Cambridge, MA: Harvard University Press.

Davis, K. (1969) *Discretionary Justice: A Preliminary Enquiry.* Baton Rouge, LA: Louisiana State University Press.

Davis, P., Lay-Yee, R., Schug, S. et al. (2001) Adverse events regional feasibility study: methodological results, *New Zealand Medical Journal,* 114(1131): 200–2.

DHSS (Department of Health and Social Security) (1966) *Health Memorandum (HM (66) 15)*. London: DHSS.

DHSS (Department of Health and Social Security) (1969) *Report of the Committee of Inquiry into Allegations of Ill-treatment of Patients and Other Irregularities at the Ely Hospital, Cardiff*, Cmnd 3975. London: HMSO.

DHSS (Department of Health and Social Security) (1971) *Report of the Fairleigh Hospital Committee of Inquiry*, Cmnd 4557. London: HMSO.

DHSS (Department of Health and Social Security) (1972) *Report of the Committee of Inquiry into Whittingham Hospital*, Cmnd 4861. London: HMSO.

DHSS (Department of Health and Social Security) (1973) *Report of the Committee on Hospital Complaints Procedure* (the Davies Committee). London: HMSO.

DHSS (Department of Health and Social Security) (1976) *NHS Code of Practice for Handling Suggestions and Complaints other than those about Family Practitioner Services*. London: DHSS.

DHSS (Department of Health and Social Security) (1978a) *The Normansfield Hospital Enquiry*, Cmnd 7357. London: HMSO.

DHSS (Department of Health and Social Security) (1978b) *Health Note (HN(78)39)*. London: DHSS.

DHSS (Department of Health and Social Security) (1981) *Health Circular (HC(81)5)*. London: DHSS.

DHSS (Department of Health and Social Security) (1983a) *NHS Management Enquiry* (The Griffiths Report). London: DHSS.

DHSS (Department of Health and Social Security) (1983b) *Press Release – More Open Complaints Procedures*. London: DHSS.

DHSS (Department of Health and Social Security) (1988) *Health Circular (HC(88)37)*. London: DHSS

Dickens, B, (1990) Wrongful birth and life, wrongful death before birth, and wrongful law, in S. McLean (ed.) *Legal Issues in Human Reproduction*. Aldershot: Dartmouth.

Dingwall, R. (1994) Litigation and the threat to medicine, in J. Gabe, D. Kelleher and G. Williams (eds) *Challenging Medicine*. London: Routledge.

Dingwall, R., Rafferty, A.M. and Webster, C. (1988) *An Introduction to the Social History of Nursing*. London: Routledge.

Dodier, N. (1994) Expert medical decisions in occupational medicine: a sociological analysis of medical judgement, *Sociology of Health and Illness*, 16(4): 488–514.

DoH (Department of Health) (1989) *Working for Patients*. London: DoH.

DoH (Department of Health) (1994) *Being Heard: The Report of a Review Committee on NHS Complaints Procedures*. London: DoH.

DoH (Department of Health) (1997) *The New NHS: Modern, Dependable*, Cm. 387. London: HMSO.

DoH (Department of Health) (1998) *A First Class Service: Quality in the New NHS*. London: HMSO.

DoH (Department of Health) (2000a) *The Report of the Inquiry into Quality and Practice Within the NHS Arising from the Actions of Rodney Ledward*, www.doh.gov.uk/stheast.

DoH (Department of Health) (2000b) *An Organisation with a Memory*. London: DoH.

DoH (Department of Health) (2001) *Handling Complaints: Monitoring the NHS Complaints Procedures, England 2000–01*, www.doh.gov.uk/nhscomplaints.

DoH (Department of Health) (2002) www.doh.gov.uk/nhscomplaints.

Donaldson, L. and Cavanagh, J. (1992) Clinical complaints and their handling: a time for change? *Quality and Regulation in Healthcare*, 1(1): 21–5.

Donnelly, M. (1997) The injury of parenthood: the tort of wrongful conception, *Northern Ireland Legal Quarterly*, 48(1): 10–23.

Ennis, M. and Grudzinskas, J. (1993) The effect of accidents and litigation on doctors, *Medical Accidents*. Oxford: Oxford Medical Publications.

Ennis, M. and Vincent, C. (1994) The effects of medical accidents and litigation on doctors and patients, *Law and Policy*, 16(2): 97–122.

Ennis, M., Clark, A. and Grudzinskas, J.G. (1991) Change in obstetric practice in response to fear of litigation in the British Isles, *The Lancet*, 338: 616–18.

Erichsen, M. (2001) The Danish patient insurance system, *Medicine and Law*, 20: 355–69.

Felstiner, W., Abel, R. and Sarat, A. (1980–1) The emergence and transformation of disputes: naming, blaming, claiming, *Law and Society Review*, 15: 631–54.

Fiss, O.M. (1984) Against settlement, *Yale Law Journal*, 93: 1073–90.

Fitzgerald, J. and Dickens, R. (1980–1) Disputing in legal and non-legal contexts: some questions for sociologists of law, *Law and Society Review*, 15(3–4): 681–706.

Fitzpatrick, R. (1991) Surveys of patient satisfaction: I – Important general considerations, *British Medical Journal*, 302: 887–9.

Fitzpatrick, R. (1993) Scope and measurement of patient satisfaction, in R. Fitzpatrick and A. Hopkins (eds), *Measurement of Patients' Satisfaction with their Care*. London: Royal College of Physicians.

Fitzpatrick, R. and Hopkins, A. (1983) Problems in the conceptual framework of patients satisfaction research: an empirical exploration, *Sociology of Health and Illness*, 5(3): 297–311.

Flynn, R. (1991) Coping with cutbacks and managing retrenchment in health, *Journal of Social Policy*, 20(2): 215–36.

Foucault, M. (1973) *The Birth of the Clinic*. London: Tavistock.

Fox, R. (1957) Training for uncertainty, in R. Merton, G. Reader and P. Kendall (eds) *The Student Physician*. Cambridge, MA: Harvard University Press.

Freidson, E. (1980) *Doctoring Together: A Study of Professional Social Control*. Chicago: University of Chicago Press.

Fuller, L. (1978) The forms and limits of adjudication, *Harvard Law Review*, 92: 353–403.

Galanter, M. (1983) The radiating effects of the courts, in K. Boyum and L. Mather (eds) *Empirical Theories about Courts*. New York: Longman.

Gawande, A.A., Thomas, E.J. and Brennan, T.A. (1999) The incidence and nature of adverse events in Colorado and Utah, *Surgery*, 126(1): 66.

Geffen, T. (1990) The complaints procedure, *Health Trends*, 22: 2.

Genn, H. and Lloyd-Bostock, S. (1995) *Medical Negligence Research Project: The Operation of the Tort System in Medical Negligence Cases*, final report to the Nuffield Foundation. London: Nuffield Foundation.

Giddens, A. (1991) *Modernity and Self-identity: Self and Society in the Late Modern Age*. Cambridge: Polity Press.

Gill, D. (1971) The British National Health Service: professional determinants of administrative structure, *International Journal of Health Services*, 1(4): 341–53.

Gilly, M., Stevenson, W. and Yale, L. (1991) Dynamics of complaint management in the service organisation, *Journal of Consumer Affairs*, winter: 295–322.

GMC (General Medical Council) (1998) *Good Medical Practice*. London: GMC.

GMC (General Medical Council) (2002) www.gmc.org.

Goffman, E. (1971) *The Presentation of Self in Everyday Life*. London: Pelican Books.

Goffman, I. (1961) *Encounters: Two Studies in the Sociology of Interaction*. Indianapolis, IN: Bobbs-Merrill.

Goffman, I. (1967) *Interaction Ritual: Essays on Face-to-Face Behaviour*. New York: Doubleday.

Habermas, J. (1976) *Legitimation Crisis*. London: Heinemann.

Ham, C. (1992) *Health Policy in Britain – The Politics and Organisation of the NHS*. London: Macmillan.

Ham, C., Dingwall, R., Fenn, P. and Harris, D. (1988) *Medical Negligence: Compensation and Accountability*. Oxford: Centre for Socio-Legal Studies.

Harlow, C. and Rawlings, R. (1998) *Law and Administration*. London: Butterworth.

Harper Mills, D. and von Bolschwing, G. (1995) Clinical risk management: experiments from the US, *Quality in Health Care*, 4(2): 90–101.

Harpwood, V. (1994) Medical negligence claims and NHS complaints, *Professional Negligence*, 10(3): 74–81.

Harris, D., Maclean, M., Genn, H. et al. (1984) *Compensation and Support for Illness and Injury*. Oxford: Clarendon Press.

Harrison, S. and Pollitt, C. (1994) *Controlling Health Professionals: The Future of Work and Organization in the NHS*. Buckingham: Open University Press.

Harrison, S., Hunter, D. and Pollitt, C. (1990) *The Dynamics of British Health Policy*. London: Unwin Hyman.

Haug, M. (1973) Deprofessionalisation: an alternative hypothesis for the future, in P. Halmos (ed.) *Professionalisation and Social Change (Sociological Review Monograph 20)*. Keele: University of Keele.

Haug, M. (1988) A re-examination of the hypothesis of deprofessionalisation, *The Millbank Quarterly*, 66(2): 48–56.

Haug, M. and Lavin, B. (1983) *Consumerism in Medicine: Challenging Physician Authority*. Beverley Hills, CA: Sage.

Hawkins, K., (1992) The uses of legal discretion: perspectives from law and social science, in K. Hawkins (ed.) *The Uses of Discretion*. Oxford: Clarendon Press.

HCSA (Hospital Consultants and Specialists Association) (2002) www.hcsa.com.

Hiatt, H., Barnes, B., Brennan, T. et al. (1989) A study of medical injury and medical malpractice: an overview, *New England Journal of Medicine*, 321: 480–4.

Hickson, G., Clayton, E., Gitnens, P. and Sloan, F. (1992) Factors that prompted families to file medical malpractice claims following perinatal injuries, *Journal of the American Medical Association*, 267(16): 1359–63.

Higgins, J. (2001) Adverse events or patterns of failure? *British Journal of Health Care Management*, 7(4): 145.

Hoffenberg, R. (1995) Foreword, in M. Rosenthal (ed.) *The Incompetent Doctor*. Buckingham: Open University Press.

Hopkins, A (1993) The doctor's perspective, in R. Fitzpatrick and A. Hopkins (eds) *Measurement of Patients' Satisfaction with their Care*, pp. 99–114. London: Royal College of Physicians.

House of Commons (1999) *Health Committee's Sixth Report: Procedures Relating to Adverse Clinical Incidents and Outcomes in Medical Care*. London: The Stationery Office.

Hoyte, P. (1998) Independent reviews in general practice – the story so far? *The Journal of the Medical Defence Union*, 14(2): 14–16.

HSC (Health Service Commissioner) (1996–7) *Annual Report*. London: HMSO.

HSC (Health Service Commissioner) (1997–8) *Annual Report*. London: HMSO.

HSC (Health Service Commissioner) (1998–9) *Annual Report*. London: HMSO.

HSC (Health Service Commissioner) (1999–2000) *Annual Report*. London: HMSO.

HSC (Health Service Commissioner) (2000–1) *Annual Report*. London: HMSO.

Hunt, H. (1991) Consumer satisfaction, dissatisfaction, and complaining behavior, *Journal of Social Issues*, 1: 107–17.

Hunter, D. (2000) *The Politics of the NHS*. London: Routledge.

Hutter, B. (1988) *The Reasonable Arm of the Law? The Law Enforcement Procedures of Environmental Health Officers*. Oxford: Clarendon Press.

Ison, T. (1997) Administrative justice – is it such a good idea? Paper presented at the Bristol Administrative Justice Conference.

Jain, O. and Ogden, J. (1999) GPs' experiences of patients' complaints: qualitative study, *British Medical Journal*, 318: 1596.

Jost, T., Mulcahy, L., Strasser, S. and Sachs, L. (1993) Consumers, complaints and professional discipline: a look at medical licensure boards, *Health Matrix: Case Western Reserve University Journal of Law and Medicine*, spring: 309–38.

Kadzombe, A. and Coals, J. (1992) Complaints against doctors in an accident and emergency department: a ten year analysis, *Archives of Emergency Medicine*, 9: 134–42.

Kagan, R.A. (1984) Inside administrative law, *Columbia Law Review*, 84: 816–32.

Kahn, P. (1999) *The Cultural Study of Law: Reconstructing Legal Scholarship*. Chicago: University of Chicago Press.

Kaye, C. and MacManus, T. (1990) Understanding complaints, *Health Service Journal*, 1990: 1254–5.

Kelleher, D., Gabe, J. and Williams, G. (1994) Understanding medical dominance in the modern world, in J. Gabe, D. Kelleher and G. Williams (eds) *Challenging Medicine*. London: Routledge.

Kennedy, I. and Grubb, A. (2000) *Medical Law: Text with Materials*. London: Butterworths.

Klein, R. (1989) *The Politics of the NHS*, 2nd edn. London: Longman.

Kolb, D.M. (1987) Corporate ombudsmen and organization conflict review, *Journal of Conflict Resolution*, 31: 673–91.

Krizek, T.J. (2000) Surgical error: ethical issues of adverse events, *Archives of Surgery*, 135(11): 1359–66.

Kyffin, R., Cook, G. and Jones, M. (1997) *Complaints Handling and Monitoring in the NHS: A Study of 12 Trusts in the North West Region*. Liverpool: University of Liverpool Institute of Medicine, Law and Bioethics.

Ladinsky, J. and Susmilch, C. (1983) Community Factors in the Brokerage of Consumer Product and Service Problems, Working Paper No. 14. Madison, WI: Wisconsin University.

Lavery, P. (1988) The physician's reaction to a malpractice suit, *Obstetrics and Gynaecology*, 70: 138–41.

Leape, L. (1999) Error in medicine, in M. Rosenthal, L. Mulcahy and S. Lloyd-Bostock (eds) *Medical Mishaps: Pieces of the Puzzle*. Buckingham: Open University Press.

Leape, L., Brennan, T., Laird, N. et al. (1991) Incidence of adverse events in hospitalised patients: results of the Harvard Medical Malpractice Study II, *New England Journal of Medicine*, 324: 377–84.

Lewis, N. and Birkinshaw, P. (1993) *When Citizens Complain: Reforming Justice and Administration*. Buckingham: Open University Press.

Lewis, N., Seneviratne, M. and Cracknell, S. (1987) Complaints Procedures in Local Government. Unpublished document, Centre for Criminological and Socio-Legal Studies, University of Sheffield.

Linder-Pelz, S. (1982) Social psychological determinants of patient satisfaction: a test of five hypotheses, *Social Science and Medicine*, 16: 583–9.

Lindgren, O.H., Christensen, R. and Harper Mills, D. (1991) Medical malpractice risk management early warning systems, *Law and Contemporary Problems*, 54(2): 23–41.

Linnea Schneid, T. (1994) An explication of treatment ideology among mental health care providers, *Sociology of Health and Illness*, 16(5): 668–93.

Littlewood, R. and Lipsedge, M. (1989) *Aliens and Alienists: Ethnic Minorities and Psychiatry*. London: Routledge.

Lloyd-Bostock, S. (1992) Attributions and apologies in letters of complaint in hospitals and letters of response, in J. Harvey, T. Orbach and A. Weber (eds) *Attribution, Accounts and Close Relationships*. New York: Springer Verlag.

Lloyd-Bostock, S. (1999) Calling doctors and hospitals to account: complaining and claiming as social processes, in M. Rosenthal, L. Mulcahy and S. Lloyd-Bostock (eds) *Medical Mishaps – Pieces of the Puzzle*. Buckingham: Open University Press.

Lloyd-Bostock, S. and Mulcahy, L. (1994) The social psychology of making and responding to hospital complaints: an account model of complaint processes, *Law and Policy*, 16: 123–47.

Locker, D. and Dunt, D. (1978) Theoretical and methodological issues in sociological studies of consumer satisfaction with medical care, *Social Science and Medicine*, 12: 283–92.

Longley, D. (1993) *Public Law and Health Service Accountability*. Buckingham: Open University Press.

Lord Chancellor's Department (1996) *Access to Justice*. London: HMSO.

Lupton, D. (1997) Doctors on the medical profession, *Sociology of Health and Illness*, 19(4): 480–97.

Macaulay, S. (1963) Non-contractual relations in business, *American Sociological Review*, 28: 55–123.

MacDonald, K. (1995) *The Sociology of the Professions*. London: Sage.

Macfarlane, A. and Chamberlain, G. (1993) What is happening to caesarean section rates? *The Lancet*, 342: 1005–6.

MacIntyre, S. and Oldman, K. (1977) Coping with migraine, in A. Davies and G. Horobin (eds) *Medical Encounters*. London: Croom Helm.

Marcantonio, E.R., McKean, S. and Brennan, T.A. (1999) Factors associated with unplanned hospital readmission among patients 80 years of age and older in a Medicare managed care plan, *The American Journal of Medicine*, 107(1): 13.

Mason, J. and McCall-Smith, R. (1994) *Law and Medical Ethics*, 4th edn. London: Butterworths.

Mather, L. and Yngvesson, B. (1980–1) Language, audience, and the transformation of disputes, *Law and Society Review*, 15(3–4): 775–821.

May, A. (1991) Aggrieved patients' journeys to justice: self-help networks among suers and non-suers. Paper presented at the Law and Society Conference, Amsterdam.

May, A. (1998) Take it up with the kipper, *Health Service Journal*, 1 October.

May, A. and Stengel, D.B. (1987) Who sues their doctors? How patients handle medical grievances, *Law and Society Review*, 124(1): 104–20.

May, M. and DeMarco, L. (1986) Patients and Doctors Disputing: Patients' Complaints and What They Do About Them, Working Paper Series 7. Chicago: Disputes Processing Research Program.

McAuslan, P. (1985) Dicey and his influence on public law, *Public Law*, 1994: 721.

McIlwain, J. (2001) A conceptual approach for the rapid reporting of clinical incidents: a proposal for benchmarking, *Clinician in Management*, 10(3): 153–9.

McIntyre, N. and Popper, K. (1989) Theoretical attitude in medicine: the need for a new ethics, *British Medical Journal*, 287: 1919–23.

McKinlay, J. and Stoekl, J. (1988) Corporatization and the social transformation of doctoring, *International Journal of Health Services*, 18(2): 191–205.

McNair-Wilson, M. (1989) Private interview with the author at the House of Commons.

McQuade, J.S. (1991) The medical malpractice crisis – reflections on the alleged caused and proposed cures: discussion paper, *Journal of the Royal Society of Medicine*, 84: 408–11.

Menkel-Meadow, C. (1996) Will managed care give us access to justice? in R. Smith (ed.) *Achieving Civil Justice: Appropriate Dispute Resolution for the 1990s*. London: Legal Action Group.

Merry, A. and McCall Smith, A. (2001) *Errors, Medicine and the Law*. Cambridge: Cambridge University Press.

Miller, R. and Sarat, A. (1980–1) Grievances, claims, and disputes: assessing the adversary culture, *Law and Society Review*, 15(3–4): 536–66.

Ministry of Health (1967) *First Report of the Joint Working Party on the Organisation of Work in Hospitals* (The Cogwheel Report). London: HMSO.

Mishler, E. (1984) *The Discourse of Medicine: Dialects of Medical Interviews*. Norwood, NJ: Ablex Publishing.

Mizrahi, T. (1984) Managing medical mistakes: ideology, insularity and account-ability among internists in training, *Social Science and Medicine*, 19: 135–46.

Mnookin, R. and Kornhauser, L. (1979) Bargaining in the shadow of the law: the case of divorce, *Yale Law Journal*, 88: 950–78.

Moore, A. (2000) Doctors launch professional and personal attack on GMC, *Health Service Journal*, 8 June: 6.

Moore, S.F. (1995) Imperfect communications, in P. Caplan (ed.) *Understanding Disputes: The Politics of Argument*. Oxford: Berg.

MORI (Market and Opinion Research Institute) (1995) *Attitudes Towards and Experiences of Complaints Systems*. London: HMSO.

MORI (Market and Opinion Research Institute) (1997) *Complaint Handling: 1997 Report*. London: MORI.

Moss, J. and Stacey, M. (1994) Analysis of evidence submitted to the Wilson Committee prepared for the House of Commons Select Committee on Health. Unpublished document.

Mulcahy, L. (1999) Patient orientated approaches to dealing with medical negligence claims, in M. Rosenthal, L. Mulcahy and S. Lloyd-Bostock (eds) *Medical Mishaps: Pieces of the Puzzle*. Buckingham: Open University Press.

Mulcahy, L. (2000) From fear to fraternity: a socio-legal analysis of doctors' responses to being called to account. Unpublished PhD thesis, London: University of North London.

Mulcahy, L. and Allsop, J. (1997) A Woolf in sheep's clothing? The move to informalism in NHS tribunals, in P. Leyland and T. Woods (eds) *Administrative Law: Facing the Future.* London: Blackstone.

Mulcahy, L. and Lloyd-Bostock, S. (1992) Complaining – what's the use? in R. Dingwall and P. Fenn (eds) *Quality in Health Care.* London: Routledge.

Mulcahy, L. and Lloyd-Bostock, S. (1994) Managers as third-party dispute handlers in complaints about hospitals, *Law and Policy*, 16(2): 185–208.

Mulcahy, L. and Rosenthal, M. (1999) Beyond blaming and perfection: a multi-dimensional approach to medical mishap, in M. Rosenthal, L. Mulcahy and S. Lloyd-Bostock (eds) *Medical Mishaps: Pieces of the Puzzle.* Buckingham: Open University Press.

Mulcahy, L. and Tritter, J. (1998) Pathways, pyramids and icebergs? Mapping the links between dissatisfaction and complaints, *Sociology of Health and Illness*, 20(6): 823–45.

Mulcahy, L., Allsop, J. and Shirley, C. (1996a) *The Voices of Complainants and GPs in Complaints about Health Care* (Social science research papers): London: South Bank University.

Mulcahy, L., Lickiss, R., Allsop, J. and Karn, V. (1996b) *Small Voices, Big Issues: An Annotated Bibliography of the Literature on Public Sector Complaints.* London: University of North London Press.

Mulcahy, L. with Selwood, M., Summerfield, L. and Netten, A. (1999) *Mediating Medical Negligence Claims: An Option for the Future?* London: The Stationery Office.

Nader, L. (ed.) (1980) *No Access to Law: Alternatives to the American Judicial System.* New York: Academic Press.

Nathanson, V. (1999) Medical mistakes: a view from the British Medical Association, in M. Rosenthal, L. Mulcahy and S. Lloyd-Bostock (eds) *Medical Mishaps: Pieces of the Puzzle.* Buckingham: Open University Press.

National Audit Office (2001) *Handling Clinical Negligence Claims in England.* Norwich: The Stationery Office.

National Consumer Council (1994) *Getting it Right for Consumers.* London: NCC.

National Consumer Council (1999) *Self-regulation of Professionals in Health Care: Consumer Issues.* London: NCC.

Nettleton, S. and Harding, G. (1994) Protesting patients: a study of complaints submitted to a family health service authority, *Sociology of Health and Illness*, 16(1): 38–61.

NHSE (1994) *Being Heard: Report of the Review Committee on NHS Complaint Procedures.* Leeds: National Health Service Executive Committee.

NHSE (National Health Service Executive) (1996) *Complaints Listening . . . Acting . . . Improving.* London: Department of Health.

O'Neill, O. (2002) *A Question of Trust.* Cambridge: Cambridge University Press.

Oakley, A. (1980) Doctor knows best, in M. Robinson (ed.) *Women Confined.* Oxford: Blackwell.

Owen, C. (1991) Formal complaints against general practitioners: a study of a thousand cases, *British Journal of General Practice*, March.

Parry, N. and Parry, J. (1976) *The Rise of the Medical Profession*. London: Croom Helm.

Partington, M. (1997) Administrative justice 40 years after Franks: past achievements and future prospects. Paper presented at the Bristol Administrative Justice Conference.

Perkin, E. (1996) *The Rise of Professional Society – England Since 1880*. London: Routledge.

Petersen, A. and Waddell, C. (eds) (1998) *Health Matters: A Sociology of Illness, Prevention and Care*. St Leonards, NSW: Allen & Unwin.

Posnett, J., Jowett, S. and Barnett, P. (2001) *NHS Complaint Procedure National Evaluation*. London: Department of Health.

Prescott-Clarke, P. et al. (1989) *Focus on Health Care*. London: Royal Institute of Public Administration and Social Community Planning Research.

Richman, J. (1987) *Medicine and Health*. Harlow: Longman.

Ridgway, D. (1999) No fault vaccine insurance: lesson from the National Vaccine Compensation Program, *Journal of Health Policy and Law*, 24: 59–86.

Roberts, R., Pascoe, G. and Attkisson, C. (1983) Relationship of service satisfaction to life satisfaction and perceived well-being, *Evaluation and Program Planning*, 6: 373–83.

Robinson, J. (1999) The price of deceit: the reflections of an advocate, in M. Rosenthal, L. Mulcahy and S. Lloyd-Bostock (eds), *Medical Mishaps: Pieces of the Puzzle*. Buckingham: Open University Press.

Roghmann, K., Hengst, A. and Zastowny, T. (1979) Satisfaction with medical care: its measurement and relation to utilization, *Medical Care*, 17(5): 461–76.

Rosenthal, D., Marshall, V., Macpherson, A. and French, S. (1980) *Nurses, Patients and Families*. London: Croom Helm.

Rosenthal, M. (1995) *The Incompetent Doctor: Behind Closed Doors*. Buckingham: Open University Press.

Rosenthal, M. (1999) How doctors think about medical mishaps, in M. Rosenthal, L. Mulcahy and S. Lloyd-Bostock (eds) *Medical Mishaps: Pieces of the Puzzle*. Buckingham: Open University Press.

Rosenthal, M., Mulcahy, L. and Lloyd-Bostock, S. (eds) (1999) *Medical Mishaps: Pieces of the Puzzle*. Buckingham: Open University Press.

Sainsbury, R. (1994) Internal reviews and the weakening of social security claimants' rights of appeal, in G. Richardson and H. Genn (eds) *Administrative Law and Government Action – The Courts and Alternative Mechanisms of Review*. Oxford: Oxford University Press.

Saks, M. (1994) The alternatives to medicine, in J. Gabe, D. Kelleher and G. Williams (eds) *Challenging Medicine*. London: Routledge.

Salter, B. (1998) *The Politics of Change in the NHS*. Basingstoke: Macmillan.

Savage, R. and Armstrong, D. (1990) Effect of general practitioners' consulting style on patients' satisfaction: a controlled study, *British Medical Journal*, 301: 968–70.

Schimmel, E. (1964) The hazards of hospitalization, *Ann Intern Med*, 60: 100–10.

Schutz, A. (1964) The well-informed citizen: an essay on the social distribution of knowledge, in A. Brotherson (ed.) *Collected Papers*, vol. 2. The Hague: Martinus Nijhoff.

Scott, M. and Lyman, S. (1968) Accounts, *American Sociological Review*, 33(2): 309–18.

Scottish Management Executive (1994) *Being Heard: The Report of a Review Committee on NHS Complaints Procedures*. Leeds: Department of Health.

Select Committee (1977–8) *Report on the Parliamentary Commissioner*. London: HMSO.

Seneviratne, M. (1994) *Ombudsmen in the Public Sector*. Buckingham: Open University Press.

Seneviratne, M. and Cracknell, S. (1988) Consumer complaints in public sector services, *Public Administration*, 66: 181–93.

Sharpe, V. and Faden, A. (1998) *Medical Harm: Historical, Conceptual and Ethical Dimensions of Iatrogenic Illness*. Cambridge: Cambridge University Press.

Sheikh, A. and Hurwitz, B. (2001) Setting up a database of medical error in general practice: conceptual and methodological considerations, *British Journal of General Practice*, 51(462): 57–60.

Simanowitz, A. (1999) The patient's perspective, in M. Rosenthal, L. Mulcahy and S. Lloyd-Bostock (eds) *Medical Mishaps: Pieces of the Puzzle*. Buckingham: Open University Press.

Smith, R. (1994) *Medical Discipline: The Professional Conduct of the GMC 1858–1990*. Oxford: Oxford University Press.

Smith, R. (1999) Preface, in M. Rosenthal, L. Mulchay and S. Lloyd-Bostock (eds) *Medical Mishaps: Pieces of the Puzzle*. Buckingham: Open University Press.

Stacey, M. (1988) *The Sociology of Health and Healing*. London: Unwin Hyman.

Stacey, M. (1992) *Regulating British Medicine*. London: Wiley.

Stacey, M. (1999) Opening address, the Public Law Project Complaints Forum, New Connaught Rooms, London, 25 March.

Stacey, M. and Moss, P. (1996) *An Analysis of Evidence Submitted to the Wilson Committee on Hospital Complaints*. Warwick: University of Warwick.

Steele, E. (1977) Two approaches to contemporary dispute behaviour and consumer problems, *Law and Society Review*, 11(4): 667–77.

Stelling, J. and Bucher, R. (1973) Vocabularies of realism in professional socialisation, *Social Science and Medicine*, 7: 661–75.

Stimson, G. and Webb, B. (1975) *Going to See the Doctor: The Consultation Process in General Practice*. London: Routledge & Kegan Paul.

Strasser, S. and Davis, R. (1991) *Measuring Patient Satisfaction for Improved Patient Services*. Ann Arbor, MI: The Health Administration Press.

Strong, P. (1983) The rivals, in R. Dingwall and P. Lewis (eds) *The Sociology of the Professions*. London: Macmillan.

Strong, P. and Davis, A. (1977) Roles, role formats and medical encounters, *Sociological Review*, 25(4): 775–800.

Studdert, D. and Brennan, T. (2001) Toward a workable model of 'no fault' compensation for medical injury in the United States, *American Journal of Law and Medicine*, 27: 225–52.

Summerton, N. (1995) Positive and negative factors in defensive medicine: a questionnaire study of general practitioners, *British Medical Journal*, 310: 27–9.

Tedeschi, J. and Reiss, M. (1981) Verbal strategies in impression management, in C. Antaki and N. Fielding (eds) *The Psychology of Ordinary Explanations in Social Behaviour*. London: Academic Press.

Teff, H. (1994) *Reasonable Care: Legal Perspectives on the Doctor-Patient Relationship*. Oxford: Clarendon Press.

Tennen, H. and Affleck, G. (1990) Blaming others for threatening events, *Psychological Bulletin*, 108(2): 209–32.

Thomas, E. and Brennan, T. (2000) Incidence and types of preventable adverse events in elderly patients: population based review of medical records, *British Medical Journal*, 320: 741–4.

Thompson, A. (1993) Inpatients: opinions of the quality of acute hospital care: discrimination as the key to measurement validity, in R. Fitzpatrick and A. Hopkins (eds) *Measurement of Patients' Satisfaction with their Care*, pp. 19–32. London: Royal College of Physicians.

Toombs, K. (1992) *The Meaning of Illness – A Phenomenological Account of the Different Perspectives of Physician and Patient*. Norwell, MA: Kluwer Academic Publishers.

Truelove, A. (1985) On handling complaints, *Hospital and Health Services Review*, September: 229–31.

Vincent, C. (1995) *Clinical Risk Management*. London: BMJ.

Vincent, C., Pincus, T. and Scurr, J. (1993) Patients' experience of surgical accidents, *Quality in Health Care*, 2: 77–82.

Vincent, C., Young, M. and Phillips, A. (1994) Why do people sue doctors? A study of patients and relatives taking legal action, *The Lancet*, 343: 1609–13.

Wallace, H. and Mulcahy, L. (1999) *Cause for Complaint: An Evaluation of the Effectiveness of the NHS Complaints Procedure*. London: Public Law Project.

Watson, S. (Secretary of the Joint Consultants Committee) (1992) Private interview.

Weeks, J. (1995) *Inventing Moralities: Sexual Values in an Age of Uncertainty*. Cambridge: Polity Press.

Weiner, B., Frieze, I., Kukla, A. et al. (1972) Perceiving the causes of success and failure, in E. Jones et al. (eds) *Attribution: Perceiving and Causes of Behaviour*. Tenson, NJ: General Learning Press.

Whetten-Goldstein, K., Kulas, E., Sloan, F., Hickson, G. and Entman, S. (1999) Compensation for birth related injury – no fault programs compared with tort, *Archive of Pediatric and Adolescent Medicine*, 153: 41–8.

Willcocks, A. (1967) *The Creation of the NHS: A Study of Pressure Groups and a Major Social Policy Decision*. London: Routledge.

Williams, B., Coyle, J. and Healy, D. (1998) The meaning of patient satisfaction and explanation of high reported levels, *Social Science and Medicine*, 47(9): 1361–71.

Williams, G. and Popay, J. (1994) Lay knowledge and the privilege of experience, in J. Gabe, D. Kelleher and G. Williams (eds) *Challenging Medicine*. London: Routledge.

Wilson, D.G., Runciman, W.B., Gibberd, R.W. et al. (1995) The Quality in Australian Health Care Study, *Medical Journal of Australia*, 163: 485–71.

Wu, A., Folkman, S., McPhee, J. and Lo, B. (1991) Do house officers learn from their mistakes? *Journal of the American Medical Association*, 265: 16–24.

Index

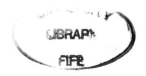

KEY CONCEPTS AND DEBATES IN HEALTH AND SOCIAL POLICY

Nigel Malin, Stephen Wilmot and Jill Manthorpe

This book identifies key social policy concepts and explores their relevance for health and welfare policy, and for the practice of professionals such as nurses and social workers who are involved in the delivery of services and provision. The text adopts ideologies of welfare approach using examples of recent policy shifts to illustrate theoretical and political tensions. This shift in emphasis away from the traditional approach of documenting policy areas is an important feature of the book. The concepts are organized in terms of doctrinal contests. This allows the authors to explore the tension between different approaches and ways of defining social policy. The aim is to help professionals identify these tensions, to be aware of the strategic choices which have been made in national and agency policy, and to locate their own practice in relationship to these choices. It draws upon the continuing debate around the Third Way and New Labour policies as they apply to health and social welfare; and identifies tensions within a non-ideological, pragmatic set of practices.

Key Concepts and Debates in Health and Social Policy has been written with students and practitioners in mind. It is a valuable resource for a wide range of health and welfare professionals, especially in nursing, social work and occupational therapy. It is also suitable for use on professional training courses, and with students of social policy and health studies.

Contents

Introduction – The Third Way: a distinct approach? – Identifying the Health Problem: need or risk? – Responsibility and Solidarity – Consumerism or Empowerment? – Central Planning and Market Competition – Controlling Service Delivery: professionalism versus managerialism – Community Care and Family Policy – Evaluating Services: quality assurance and the quality debate – Prioritizing and Rationing – Conclusion – Index.

176pp   0 335 19905 4 (Paperback)   0 335 19906 2 (Hardback)

REGULATING HEALTHCARE
A PRESCRIPTION FOR IMPROVEMENT?

Kieran Walshe

Healthcare organizations in the UK and the USA face a growing tide of regulation, accreditation, inspection and external review, aimed at improving their performance. In the USA, over three decades of healthcare regulation by state and federal government and by non-governmental agencies have created a complex, costly and overlapping network of oversight arrangements for healthcare organizations. In the UK's government run National Health Service, regulation is central to current health policy, with the creation of a host of new national agencies and inspectorates tasked with overseeing the performance of NHS hospitals and other organizations.

But does regulation work? This book:

- explores the development and use of healthcare regulation in both countries, comparing and contrasting their experience and drawing on regulatory research in other industries and settings
- offers a structured approach to analysing what regulators do and how they work
- develops principles for effective regulation, aimed at maximizing the benefits of regulatory interventions and minimizing their costs

Regulating Healthcare will be read by those with an interest or involvement in health policy and management, including policy makers, healthcare managers, health professionals and students. It is particularly suitable for use on postgraduate health and health related programmes.

Contents

Series Editor's introduction – Introduction – Regulation: concepts and theories – Regulating healthcare in the United States – Regulating healthcare in the United Kingdom – Analysing healthcare regulation – Conclusions: The future for healthcare regulation – References – Further reading – Index.

c. 224 pp   0 335 21022 8 (Paperback)   0 335 21023 6 (Hardback)